Traumatic Brain Injury: Defining Best Practice

Guest Editors

SILVANA RIGGIO, MD
ANDY JAGODA, MD, FACEP

PSYCHIATRIC CLINICS OF NORTH AMERICA

www.psych.theclinics.com

December 2010 • Volume 33 • Number 4

SAUNDERS an imprint of ELSEVIER, Inc.

W.B. SAUNDERS COMPANY
A Division of Elsevier Inc.

1600 John F. Kennedy Boulevard • Suite 1800 • Philadelphia, PA 19103-2899

http://www.theclinics.com

PSYCHIATRIC CLINICS OF NORTH AMERICA Volume 33, Number 4
December 2010 ISSN 0193-953X, ISBN-13: 978-1-4377-2492-9

Editor: Sarah E. Barth
Developmental Editor: Jessica Demetriou

© 2010 Elsevier Inc. All rights reserved.

This journal and the individual contributions contained in it are protected under copyright by Elsevier, and the following terms and conditions apply to their use:

Photocopying
Single photocopies of single articles may be made for personal use as allowed by national copyright laws. Permission of the Publisher and payment of a fee is required for all other photocopying, including multiple or systematic copying, copying for advertising or promotional purposes, resale, and all forms of document delivery. Special rates are available for educational institutions that wish to make photocopies for non-profit educational classroom use. For information on how to seek permission visit www.elsevier.com/permissions or call: (+44) 1865 843830 (UK)/(+1) 215 239 3804 (USA).

Derivative Works
Subscribers may reproduce tables of contents or prepare lists of articles including abstracts for internal circulation within their institutions. Permission of the Publisher is required for resale or distribution outside the institution. Permission of the Publisher is required for all other derivative works, including compilations and translations (please consult www.elsevier.com/permissions).

Electronic Storage or Usage
Permission of the Publisher is required to store or use electronically any material contained in this journal, including any article or part of an article (please consult www.elsevier.com/permissions). Except as outlined above, no part of this publication may be reproduced, stored in a retrieval system or transmitted in any form or by any means, electronic, mechanical, photocopying, recording or otherwise, without prior written permission of the Publisher.

Notice
No responsibility is assumed by the Publisher for any injury and/or damage to persons or property as a matter of products liability, negligence or otherwise, or from any use or operation of any methods, products, instructions or ideas contained in the material herein. Because of rapid advances in the medical sciences, in particular, independent verification of diagnoses and drug dosages should be made.

Although all advertising material is expected to conform to ethical (medical) standards, inclusion in this publication does not constitute a guarantee or endorsement of the quality or value of such product or of the claims made of it by its manufacturer.

Psychiatric Clinics of North America (ISSN 0193-953X) is published quarterly by Elsevier Inc., 360 Park Avenue South, New York, NY 10010-1710. Months of issue are March, June, September, and December. Business and Editorial Offices: 1600 John F. Kennedy Blvd., Suite 1800, Philadelphia, PA 19103-2899. Periodicals postage paid at New York, NY and additional mailing offices. Subscription prices are $265.00 per year (US individuals), $473.00 per year (US institutions), $131.00 per year (US students/residents), $321.00 per year (Canadian individuals), $589.00 per year (Canadian Institutions), $399.00 per year (foreign individuals), $589.00 per year (foreign institutions), and $194.00 per year (international & Canadian students/residents). Foreign air speed delivery is included in all *Clinics'* subscription prices. All prices are subject to change without notice. **POSTMASTER:** Send address changes to *Psychiatric Clinics of North America*, Elsevier Health Sciences Division, Subscription Customer Service, 3251 Riverport Lane, Maryland Heights, MO 63043. Customer Service: 1-800-654-2452 (US). From outside the United States, call 1-314-447-8871. Fax: 1-314-447-8029. E-mail: journalscustomerservice-usa@elsevier.com (for print support) and journalsonlinesupport-usa@elsevier.com (for online support).

Reprints. For copies of 100 or more, of articles in this publication, please contact the Commercial Reprints Department, Elsevier Inc., 360 Park Avenue South, New York, New York 10010-1710. Tel.: (212) 633-3813, Fax: (212) 462-1935, E-mail: reprints@elsevier.com.

Psychiatric Clinics of North America is covered in *MEDLINE/PubMed (Index Medicus)*, *Current Contents/Social and Behavioral Sciences, Social Science Citation Index, Embase/Excerpta Medica,* and PsycINFO.

Printed and bound by CPI Group (UK) Ltd, Croydon, CR0 4YY

Transferred to Digital Print 2012

Contributors

GUEST EDITORS

SILVANA RIGGIO, MD
Professor of Psychiatry and Neurology, Mount Sinai School of Medicine;
Director of Consultation Liaison Service, James J. Peters VAMC, New York, New York

ANDY JAGODA, MD, FACEP
Professor and Chair, Department of Emergency Medicine, Mount Sinai School
of Medicine, New York, New York

AUTHORS

CAPT(r) STEPHEN T. AHLERS, PhD
US Navy Director, Operational and Undersea Medicine Directorate, Naval Medical
Research Center, Silver Spring, Maryland

DMITRI BOUGAKOV, PhD
City University of New York, New York

JOSHUA SETH BRODER, MD, FACEP
Associate Professor, Division of Emergency Medicine, Department of Surgery,
Duke University Medical Center, Durham, North Carolina

ADAM CHODOBSKI, PhD
Associate Professor, Department of Emergency Medicine, Alpert Medical School
of Brown University, Rhode Island Hospital, Providence, Rhode Island

HELEN CORONEL, MSN, FNP
Defense and Veterans Brain Injury Center, Washington, DC

ADRIAN CRISTIAN, MD
Practice Chief, Rehabilitation Medicine Service, James J. Peters Department
of Veterans Affairs Medical Center, Bronx; Associate Professor, Department
of Rehabilitation Medicine, Mount Sinai School of Medicine, New York, New York

KRISTEN DAMS-O'CONNOR, PhD
Department of Rehabilitation Medicine, Mount Sinai School of Medicine, New York,
New York

SHANA DE CARO, Esq
De Caro & Kaplen LLP, Pleasantville, New York; Officer, Traumatic Brain Injury
Litigation Group, American Association for Justice; Trustee, Civil Justice Foundation;
Vice President, American Academy of Brain Injury Attorneys

GREGORY A. ELDER, MD
Practice Chief, Neurology Service, James J. Peters Department of Veterans Affairs
Medical Center, Bronx; Professor, Departments of Psychiatry and Neurology, Mount Sinai
School of Medicine, New York, New York

HAYLEY FIVECOAT, BS
Research Program Coordinator, Department of Neurology, Mount Sinai School
of Medicine, New York, New York

STEVEN R. FLANAGAN, MD
Professor of Rehabilitation Medicine, Rusk Institute of Rehabilitation Medicine,
New York University School of Medicine, New York, New York

KATHERINE GIFFORD, PsyD
Division of Neuropsychology, Henry Ford Health System, Detroit, Michigan

ELKHONON GOLDBERG, PhD
Clinical Professor, Department of Neurology, New York University School of Medicine,
New York, New York

WAYNE A. GORDON, PhD
Jack Nash Professor, Department of Rehabilitation Medicine; Director, Brain Injury
Research Center, Mount Sinai School of Medicine, New York, New York

LAP HO, PhD
Assistant Professor, Department of Neurology, Mount Sinai School of Medicine,
New York, New York

MICHAEL S. JAFFEE, MD
Defense and Veterans Brain Injury Center, Washington, DC

ANDY S. JAGODA, MD, FACEP
Professor and Chair, Department of Emergency Medicine, Mount Sinai School
of Medicine, New York, New York

MICHAEL V. KAPLEN, Esq
De Caro & Kaplen LLP, Pleasantville, New York; Chair, New York State Traumatic Brain
Injury Services Coordinating Council; Past Chair, Traumatic Brain Injury Litigation Group,
American Association for Justice; President, American Academy of Brain Injury Attorneys

JAIME M. LEVINE, DO
Instructor of Rehabilitation Medicine, Rusk Institute of Rehabilitation Medicine,
New York University School of Medicine, New York, New York

DONALD W. MARION, MD
Defense and Veterans Brain Injury Center, Washington, DC

KIMBERLY S. MEYER, MSN, ACNP
Defense and Veterans Brain Injury Center, Washington, DC; University of Louisville
Hospital, Trauma Institute, Louisville, Kentucky

EFFIE M. MITSIS, PhD
Assistant Professor, Department of Psychiatry, Mount Sinai School of Medicine,
New York; Neuropsychologist, Rehabilitation Medicine Service, James J. Peters
Department of Veterans Affairs Medical Center, Bronx, New York

GIULIO MARIA PASINETTI, MD, PhD
Professor, Department of Neurology, Mount Sinai School of Medicine, New York;
Geriatric Research, Education and Clinical Center, James J. Peters Veteran Affairs
Medical Center, Bronx, New York

KENNETH PODELL, PhD
Division of Neuropsychology, Henry Ford Health System; Clinical Associate Professor, Department of Psychiatry, Wayne State University, Detroit, Michigan

SILVANA RIGGIO, MD
Professor of Psychiatry and Neurology, Mount Sinai School of Medicine;
Director of Consultation Liaison Service, James J. Peters VAMC, New York, New York

JOANNA SZMYDYNGER-CHODOBSKA, PhD
Assistant Professor, Department of Emergency Medicine, Alpert Medical School of Brown University, Rhode Island Hospital, Providence, Rhode Island

BRIAN J. ZINK, MD
Professor and Chair, Department of Emergency Medicine, Alpert Medical School of Brown University, Rhode Island Hospital and The Miriam Hospital, Providence, Rhode Island

Contents

> A complex set of molecular and functional reactions is set into motion by traumatic brain injury (TBI). New research that extends beyond pathological effects on neurons suggests a key role for the blood-brain barrier, neurovascular unit, arginine vasopressin, and neuroinflammation in the pathophysiology of TBI. The prevalence of molecular derangements in TBI holds promise for the identification and use of biomarkers to assess severity of injury, determine prognosis, and perhaps direct therapy. Hopefully, improved knowledge of these elements of pathophysiology will provide the mechanistic clues that lead to improved treatment of TBI.

> Traumatic brain injury (TBI) has been a major cause of mortality and morbidity in the wars in Iraq and Afghanistan. Blast exposure has been the most common cause of TBI, occurring through multiple mechanisms. What is less clear is whether the primary blast wave causes brain damage through mechanisms that are distinct from those common in civilian TBI and whether multiple exposures to low-level blast can lead to long-term sequelae. Complicating TBI in soldiers is the high prevalence of posttraumatic stress disorder. At present, the relationship is unclear. Resolution of these issues will affect both treatment strategies and strategies for the protection of troops in the field.

> Traumatic brain injury (TBI) is a known injury in today's combat arena. Improved screening and surveillance methods have diagnosed TBI with increasing frequency. Current treatment plans are based largely on information gleaned from sports injuries. However, these management paradigms fail to address the effect of physiologic stress (fatigue, dehydration) and psychological stress at the time of injury as well as the number of previous concussions that may affect recovery from combat-related TBI. This article presents current evaluation and management of combat-related injury and discusses other psychological conditions that may coexist with TBI.

> The definition of a mild traumatic brain injury (TBI) has come under close scrutiny and is changing as a result of refined diagnostic testing. Although

up to 15% of patients with a mild TBI will have an acute intracranial lesion identified on head computed tomography (CT), less than 1% of these patients will have a lesion requiring a neurosurgical intervention. Evidence-based guideline methodology has assisted in generating recommendations to facilitate clinical decision making; however, no set of guidelines is 100% sensitive and specific. Evidence supports the safety of discharging patients with mild TBI who have a negative CT. However, though patients with a negative CT are at almost no risk of deteriorating from a neurosurgical lesion, a key intervention is to provide these patients at discharge from the emergency department with counseling regarding postconcussive symptoms, when to return to work, school, or sports, and when to seek additional medical care.

a holistic approach when assessing and treating the patient and consider the patient in total, including premorbid and post-incident factors, to formulate a comprehensive and accurate picture of the patient. This approach will guide the clinician regarding multiple types of treatment the patient may require.

Rehabilitation following traumatic brain injury (TBI) is best provided by an interdisciplinary team of health care providers that takes advantage of the unique skills of multiple specialists, as well as their combined strengths that address problems that cut across disciplines. The setting where rehabilitation is provided is determined by the medical stability of patients, their ability to tolerate intensive therapies, and their likelihood of community reintegration within a reasonable period of time. Successful rehabilitation requires prompt recognition and treatment of TBI-related medical, cognitive, and behavioral problems to promote recovery and enhance community reintegration, using a combination of rehabilitation modalities and medications.

Cognitive rehabilitation interventions are theoretically based and empirically validated treatments designed to ameliorate the cognitive, behavioral, and emotional impairments commonly experienced by individuals with traumatic brain injury (TBI). Cognitive rehabilitation can play many roles in facilitating recovery after TBI, such as improving impaired cognitive functions, increasing awareness of injury-related deficits, improving mood, facilitating vocational and community involvement, and reducing the probability of secondary disability. The considerable evidence documenting the impact of cognitive rehabilitation on improving the day-to-day function of individuals with TBI is described.

Patients who have sustained a mild traumatic brain injury (TBI) from both civilian and military populations exhibit clinical symptoms of varying severity with minimal to profound impact on their daily functioning. Although most patients make a full recovery, a subgroup of mild TBI patients develop cognitive, somatic, and neurobehavioral sequelae that generally resolve over 3 to 6 months; a smaller subgroup develop persisting symptoms. The reason why a mild TBI results in varying clinical symptoms is currently unknown. Based on evidence that microRNA species in peripheral blood mononuclear cells (PBMCs) may reflect molecular alterations in neurodegenerative disorders, it can be hypothesized that at early, preclinical phases of the disease, PBMC may provide an ideal and clinically assessable "window" into the brain. Thus, it is conceivable that changes in the expression profile of clinically accessible biological indices (biomarkers), such as microRNA in PBMC, may reflect molecular alterations following TBI that contribute to the onset and progression of TBI phenotypes including chronic traumatic encephalopathy. It is possible that the availability of TBI biomarkers may provide potential elements with clinical relevance to prevention, prognosis, and treatment of postconcussive disorders.

Shana De Caro and Michael V. Kaplen

Traumatic brain injury has received significant attention in recent years. Advances in diagnosis and management have resulted in opportunities to improve patient outcomes; however, controversies in diagnosis and management have resulted in increased interactions between the medical and legal communities. This artiolo highlights some of the areas of controversy in traumatic brain injury litigation with the hope that synchronous resolutions of both legal and medical issues will ultimately benefit patient care. It is imperative that the neuroscience community engage the legal community to facilitate an understanding of the issues and their ramifications. Proactive communication and understanding between medical and legal specialties offer the potential to maximize efficiencies in our health care and legal systems.

THE CLINICS ARE NOW AVAILABLE ONLINE!

Access your subscription at:
www.theclinics.com

Preface

Traumatic Brain Injury: Defining Best Practice

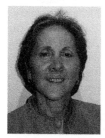 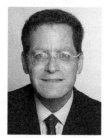

Silvana Riggio, MD   Andy Jagoda, MD
Guest Editors

Traumatic brain injury (TBI) is a complex disorder with the potential for significant long-term disability. The incidence of TBI is at epidemic proportions and rapidly growing, especially in the developing world. Not only is the incidence increasing but so is the recognition of TBI as a major health care concern. The war in Iraq and Afghanistan has resulted in an alarmingly high rate of blast exposures and research is suggesting that the blast wave is associated with injury to the central nervous system. In addition, there is growing attention from sports-related TBI, suggesting that repeat "mild" injuries may have a cumulative effect and predispose to a newly defined entity, chronic traumatic encephalopathy.

Prevention is clearly the goal, but once a TBI occurs, it requires a multidisciplinary approach to minimize injury and maximize outcomes. Outcomes from TBI are related to severity of the initial trauma and affected by comorbid conditions, and early and late interventions. Many of the long-term sequelae are behavioral and the psychiatrist often plays a key role in managing these patients. A clear understanding of the pathophysiology of TBI and the multifactorial issues that play into its acute and chronic presentations is critical. Most important, the psychiatrist is positioned to help the team differentiate the behavioral sequelae from those related to pharmacologic, medical, and structural etiologies. Indeed, in patients with primarily behavioral or neurologic sequelae from TBI, it is the psychiatrist who is perhaps best positioned to tailor a management strategy.

Management of patients who have sustained a TBI requires a team approach since the sequelae often involve multiple systems. The response to any physical or emotional disturbance is also influenced by the baseline personality structure; individual coping mechanisms; severity of the injury and its circumstances; the injury's impact on the patient's physical and intellectual functioning; and, last but not least, the social support

Psychiatr Clin N Am 33 (2010) xiii–xiv
doi:10.1016/j.psc.2010.09.005
0193-953X/10/$ – see front matter © 2010 Elsevier Inc. All rights reserved.

(or lack of). Outcomes are related to all of the preceding factors and it is imperative that they all be considered when evaluating these patients.

The concept for this issue of *Psychiatric Clinics of North America* arose from the coeditors' years of collaboration and a merger of their clinical perspectives: Silvana Riggio is a neurologist and a psychiatrist with a strong interest in frontal lobe disorders and cognitive evaluations of patients who have sustained a TBI; Andy Jagoda is an emergency physician who has focused on the acute recognition and management of TBI, and who has been involved in the development of practice guidelines for these patients. In the spirit of the multidisciplinary approach needed to care for the TBI patient, the authors recruited colleagues from a number of disciplines. An article specifically dedicated to TBI in the military is included because of its unique circumstance. Articles span the continuum of care from management in the acute phase, including neuroimaging, through cognitive assessments and neurorehabilitation.

TBI comes with an enormous cost to individuals, their families, and society. The good news is that advances have been made; however, much work remains to be done. There is a great need for improved data bases and multicenter collaborations. Perhaps the most exciting frontier in TBI research is gaining a better understanding of the neurobehavioral sequelae. New imaging technologies combined with neuropsychological and neurophysiological testing hold the potential to help identify lesions that contribute to neurobehavioral deficits that often complicate recovery. Hopefully, this issue of *Psychiatric Clinics of North America* provides the reader with a comprehensive perspective on TBI that will stimulate further research and promote quality care.

Silvana Riggio, MD
Mount Sinai School of Medicine
One Gustave L. Levy Place, Box 1230
New York, NY 10029, USA

Andy Jagoda, MD
Department of Emergency Medicine
Mount Sinai School of Medicine
One Gustave L. Levy Place, Box 1620
New York, NY 10029, USA

E-mail addresses:
silvana.riggio@mssm.edu (S. Riggio)
andy.jagoda@mssm.edu (A. Jagoda)

Emerging Concepts in the Pathophysiology of Traumatic Brain Injury

Brian J. Zink, MD[a],*, Joanna Szmydynger-Chodobska, PhD[b],
Adam Chodobski, PhD[b]

KEYWORDS

- Pathophysiology • Traumatic brain injury • TBI • ICP
- Blood-brain barrier

Traumatic brain injury (TBI) encompasses a large spectrum of pathophysiology—from the football player who is dazed after a helmet-to-helmet hit from an opponent to the motorcyclist who is comatose after crashing into a guardrail. In the mild TBI end of the spectrum, the pathological effects of concussion, which were previously not well characterized or understood, are receiving a great deal of attention in neuroscience and the media. At the other end of the spectrum, the consequences of blast injuries from explosive devices in military personnel serving in Iraq and Afghanistan have been a grim reminder that severe TBI is responsible for most of the deaths and long-term disability in people who suffer traumatic injuries.[1,2]

It is clear that a better understanding of pathophysiology from laboratory and clinical research has improved survival and outcomes from severe TBI. Better emergency medical services and emergency department care, operative intervention, intensive care, and rehabilitation have reduced the mortality in patients with severe TBI from approximately 50% in the 1970s to approximately 20% in the past decade.[1,3] This reduction in mortality has occurred without an increase in severe disability in those who survive TBI, meaning that more effective management of TBI through scientific discovery is having a positive impact across the spectrum of injury.

Effective diagnosis and care for mild TBI and concussion are currently in an evolutionary phase. New neuropsychological screening and evaluative tests and neuroimaging techniques have made it possible to identify neurological symptoms,

[a] Department of Emergency Medicine, Alpert Medical School of Brown, University Rhode Island Hospital & The Miriam Hospital, 593 Eddy Street, Claverick 2, Providence, RI 02903, USA
[b] Department of Emergency Medicine, Alpert Medical School of Brown University, Coro Center West, Room 112, 1 Hoppin Street, Providence, RI 02903, USA
* Corresponding author.
E-mail address: Brian_Zink@Brown.edu

Psychiatr Clin N Am 33 (2010) 741–756
doi:10.1016/j.psc.2010.08.005
0193-953X/10/$ – see front matter © 2010 Elsevier Inc. All rights reserved.

deficits, and pathological changes in the brain that were previously unrecognized or underappreciated.

The pathophysiology of TBI is fascinating and complex; many aspects are still not fully understood. For patients who survive the initial trauma, morbidity and mortality are largely determined by the severity of secondary injury processes, which include axonal and vascular injuries, ischemia, and the formation of cerebral edema as well as hemorrhage in or around brain tissue. An intricate cascade of molecular and functional changes occurs after injury; some of the changes are beneficial but many are harmful. The complex and interdependent nature of pathophysiological events after TBI may explain why many single-mechanism neuroprotective interventions have shown significant therapeutic potential in animal models of TBI but have failed to demonstrate consistent improvement of outcome in patients with TBI.[4] The development of combination treatments directed against multiple targets, and thus having complementary therapeutic effects, may offer the most hope for early therapy in TBI patients.[5]

Substantial work in animal models, in vitro cell culture systems, and human data suggest several factors that initiate and/or contribute to the progression of secondary injury. Many of these factors, such as release of excitatory amino acids, excessive production of free radicals, and altered calcium homeostasis, are reviewed and discussed elsewhere. This article reviews the biomechanics of TBI and considers the molecular, cellular, and functional changes that occur with a focus on dysfunction of the blood-brain barrier (BBB) and the role of neuroinflammation in the progression of injury.

BIOMECHANICS OF TBI

Brain tissue may be injured directly from traumatic forces, such as a gunshot wound or blow to the head, that fracture the skull. Many brain injuries result, however, from indirect forces that set the head, skull, and brain in motion. Forces of acceleration, deceleration, or rotation are often at play in falls, high-speed motor vehicle crashes, or, in the case of children, the shaken baby syndrome. When the skull and brain are rapidly put into motion and then stopped, inertial forces are created that can harm brain tissue. The two main inertial forces active in TBI are linear acceleration and rotational head movement. It is thought that linear acceleration forces are responsible for superficial brain lesions, whereas rotational movements may explain deeper cerebral lesions and the concussion mechanism.[6]

The tissue strains induced by both linear and rotational forces set up spatiotemporal gradients in the brain.[7] The viscoelastic properties of the brain lend little internal structural support. This makes the brain more susceptible to inertial forces and pressure gradients than more solid organs. The gray matter closest to the surface of the brain is affected by linear forces, which results in cortical contusions and hemorrhage.[8] The deeper cerebral white matter axons are more likely to be physiologically and mechanically injured by rotational forces. This alteration of deeper white matter is called diffuse axonal injury.[9] Deep gray matter nuclei and axonal tracts in the midbrain and brainstem may also be damaged by rotational forces.

Some scientists believe that the linear and rotational acceleration theories for TBI do not explain how injury to deeper cortical structures occurs in the absence of injury to more superficial cerebral structures. The stereotactile theory considers the spherical shape of the cranial vault in the setting of skull-brain relative movements and skull vibrations and the generation of secondary pressure waves. It is postulated that because brain tissue has the same density on concentric planes, the secondary waves may propagate as a spherical wave front, which focuses energy on deeper cerebral structures.[10]

After primary injury forces have unleashed their harmful effects on the brain, secondary biomechanical effects are a major factor in the eventual pathology. In the rigid skull vault, the relationship between intracranial volume and pressure is of utmost importance. As total cerebral volume increases, intracranial pressure (ICP) rises minimally at first due to autoregulation of cerebral blood flow (CBF) and the redistribution of cerebrospinal fluid (CSF). There are limits, however, to this compensation, and as cerebral volume increases more, a marked rise in ICP can occur. (**Fig. 1**) High ICP is one of the key pathologic processes in secondary injury to the brain. Brain tissue edema, hemorrhage, and hematomas all may contribute to an increase in cerebral volume, which elevates ICP.[11]

Penetrating brain injury directly injures brain tissue that is directly in the path of the projectile, but the resultant blast effect also produces significant structural damage to adjacent tissues. With penetrating injury, the trajectory and location of the wound are the most significant factors in the eventual pathology.

DYSFUNCTION OF THE BBB IN TBI

The BBB plays an essential role in maintaining an optimal microenvironment necessary for normal functioning of neurons and glia. It tightly regulates the composition of brain fluids by controlling selective access of blood-borne ions, nutrients, and

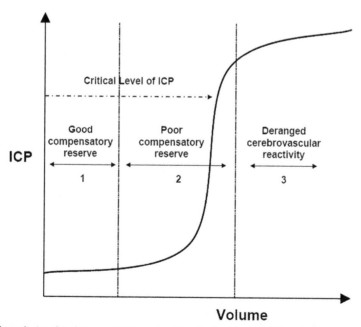

Fig. 1. The relationship between ICP and brain volume. The curve has three components: 1, normal state—good compensatory reserve; 2, increasing ICP with decreased compensatory reserve; small changes in brain volume cause proportionately larger changes in ICP; and 3, decompensated compensatory reserve—pathologically high levels of ICP occur. (*Adapted from* Smith M. Monitoring intracranial pressure in traumatic brain injury. Anesth Analg 2008;106:241; with permission.)

polypeptides to brain parenchyma. The BBB is also involved in removal of potentially noxious metabolites from brain parenchyma and prevents the entry of neurotoxic plasma constituents and xenobiotics to the central nervous system (CNS). The major anatomical components of the BBB that have a critical impact on its function are the tight junctions that connect the adjacent cerebrovascular endothelial cells forming the walls of brain microvessels. It is generally believed that the endothelial cells of parenchymal brain microvessels are not able to maintain their tight BBB phenotype by themselves and that they require the presence of astrocytes to attain these properties. It has been well documented that astrocytes, whose foot processes are intimately associated with brain endothelial cells, are crucial for maintaining the tightness of the BBB.[12] In addition to their role in long-term induction and maintenance of endothelial barrier in the CNS, astrocytes can release chemical factors that regulate various properties of the BBB, including permeability, transport activities, and endothelial interactions with circulating immune cells. Because of this close anatomical and functional relationship between the cerebrovascular endothelium and astrocytes, a new term, *the gliovascular unit*, has recently been coined.[12] Other parenchymal cells, such as pericytes, microglia, and neurons, however, are also closely associated with brain endothelium and together with astrocytes constitute the so-called neurovascular unit.[12] This newly adopted terminology reflects the complexity of anatomical and functional relations between the cerebrovascular endothelium and other parenchymal cells in the brain (**Fig. 2**).

It was not until the early 1990s that the anatomical studies of both human and animal brain tissue revealed substantial pathology associated with brain vasculature, which suggested the possible dysfunction of the BBB resulting from neurotrauma. It is now generally accepted that both traumatic and nontraumatic forms of brain injury, such as ischemic stroke and intracerebral hemorrhage, are often accompanied by dysfunction of the BBB, which is not only trigged by injury but may also affect its progression. There is a broad spectrum of pathophysiological processes involving the brain endothelium, including the loss and/or redistribution of tight junction proteins, increased permeability, augmented production of proinflammatory mediators, and changes in activity of BBB transporters, which contribute to dysfunction of the BBB.[12] There is a growing consensus that changes in function of the BBB resulting from brain injury may have a significant effect on the evolution of injury, the response to therapy, and the extent of neuronal repair.

Disruption of the BBB and the Formation of Posttraumatic Brain Edema

Cerebral edema represents an important and therapeutically difficult problem in TBI patients, particularly in moderate to severe TBI. Brain edema is also associated with other common CNS pathologies, including ischemic stroke and subarachnoid hemorrhage (SAH) or intracerebral hemorrhage. Traditionally, cerebral edema has been classified into two major categories, vasogenic edema and cytotoxic edema. Vasogenic edema is characterized by increased permeability of the BBB to low- and high-molecular-weight markers and accumulation of plasma-derived, osmotically active molecules, such as plasma proteins, in brain interstitial fluid. By comparison, cytotoxic edema is associated with changes in cell metabolism and malfunction of membrane-associated pumps and ion transporters, which result in the cellular accumulation of osmotically active molecules.

The collective effect of cytotoxic edema as millions of brain cells swell after TBI can increase cerebral volume and translate into increased tissue pressure and elevated ICP. Cytotoxic edema in neurons contributes to this process, but neurons do not constitute the majority of brain cells. Astrocytes and endothelial cells are a much

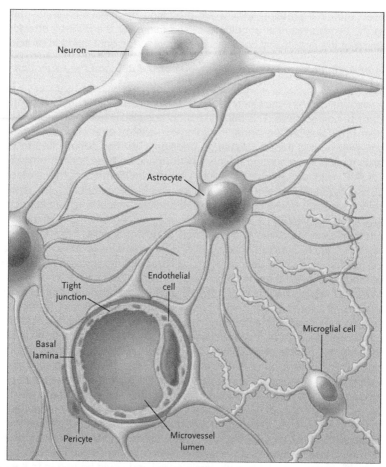

Fig. 2. The neurovascular unit. A conceptual framework, the neurovascular unit comprises neurons, the microvessels that supply them, and their supporting cells. Cerebral microvessels consist of the endothelium (which forms the BBB), the basal lamina matrix, and the end-feet of astrocytes. Microglial cells and pericytes may also participate in the unit. Communication has been shown to occur between neurons and microvessels through astrocytes. (*Reprinted from* del Zoppo GJ. Stroke and neurovascular protection. N Engl J Med 2006;354:553–5; with permission.)

greater factor in the cumulative effect of cytotoxic edema in the injured brain. Both vasogenic and cytotoxic edema are likely to be present in TBI. Animal studies have demonstrated a biphasic opening of the BBB after TBI, suggesting the formation of vasogenic edema,[13] but controversy exists as to whether or not in humans this type of edema plays an equally important role.[14]

Several factors, including reactive oxygen species (ROS), proinflammatory cytokines, vascular endothelial growth factor, and matrix metalloproteinases (MMPs), have been implicated in the leakage of the BBB observed after brain injury. Vascular endothelial growth factor, which is carried by neutrophils invading the traumatized brain parenchyma and produced by activated astrocytes, likely increases the permeability of the BBB by inducing a rapid phosphorylation and disorganization of endothelial junctional proteins. MMPs are produced by various parenchymal cells, including the cerebrovascular endothelium, and can open the BBB by attacking the basal lamina of the endothelial cells and/or degrading the tight junction proteins.

The Role of Arginine Vasopressin in Disruption of the BBB and the Formation of Cerebral Edema

Arginine vasopressin (AVP) has long been known for its role in maintaining body water and electrolyte homeostasis. This peptide hormone is also involved in the regulation of many other physiological functions, including the control of arterial blood pressure, body temperature, and insulin release. In addition, AVP has been linked to diverse mammalian social behaviors and memory performance. These various physiological actions of AVP, with the possible exception of mnemonic effects of AVP metabolites, AVP(4–9) and AVP(4–8),[15] are mediated by three known receptors, V_{1a}, V_{1b}, and V_2, of which the V_{1a} receptor (AVPR1A) is expressed on brain vasculature and astrocytes.[16] Neuronally expressed AVPR1A found in various regions of rodent and primate brains seems predominantly localized to the nucleus of neuronal cells,[16] but the functional significance of this cellular distribution of AVPR1A in neurons is currently unclear.

Several animal studies of various forms of brain injury, including TBI, cerebral ischemia, and intracerebral hemorrhage, have provided compelling evidence for the role of AVP in promoting disruption of the BBB and exacerbating the formation of cerebral edema in an injured brain. These consistent findings in diverse forms of brain injury suggest the common mechanisms that underlie these pathophysiological AVP actions; however, the nature of these mechanisms is not well understood. The data obtained in animal models of brain injury are supported by clinical observations that the levels of AVP in plasma and CSF of patients with TBI and other forms of brain injury are elevated. It also seems that, in TBI patients, the magnitude of increase of plasma concentration of AVP or copeptin, a C-terminal fragment of the AVP precursor protein, correlates with the severity of injury. Circulating AVP is predominantly produced in the paraventricular and supraoptic hypothalamic nuclei and is then released into the bloodstream within the posterior pituitary. The sources of CSF-borne AVP, however, are not obvious. It is possible that the long, AVP-containing axonal processes, which originate in the paraventricular hypothalamic nuclei and could be traced to the lateral cerebral ventricles, release AVP into the CSF.[17] It has also been discovered that the epithelium of the choroid plexus, the CSF-producing tissue located in all four cerebral ventricles, can synthesize AVP.[18]

An increase in AVP synthesis observed after brain injury is accompanied by a substantial augmentation of the expression of AVPR1A on the cerebrovascular endothelium and astrocytes.[16] The injury also results in a redistribution of this receptor from astrocyte cell bodies to astrocyte processes, which may play a role in the AVP-dependent signaling within the gliovascular/neurovascular unit. These findings are consistent with the results from animal experiments, in which the efficacy of AVPR1A antagonists in decreasing the permeability of the BBB and reducing the formation of edema in an injured brain has been demonstrated.[19,20] This suggests that interfering with AVP signaling may have beneficial therapeutic effects in TBI. The use of AVPR1A antagonists in clinical practice, however, may not always be desirable, especially in head trauma patients with multiple organ injuries, internal bleeding, and hypotension, where AVP may be a critical factor in maintaining perfusion of the brain and other vital organs.

The BBB and Drug Delivery in TBI

As discussed previously, clinical trials for neuroprotective treatments in TBI patients have provided disappointing results. One of the obstacles to the progress in translational research on TBI may be insufficient understanding of the pathophysiology of the BBB, especially with regard to changes in function of this endothelial barrier that are relevant to drug delivery to an injured brain. Although several factors, such as the perturbations in CBF and brain metabolism, as well as increased interstitial pressure, all of which may occur in TBI, have been recognized to have an impact on brain bioavailability of neuroprotective agents,[21] much less consideration has been given to possible posttraumatic changes in expression and activity of the xenobiotic transport systems that are present at the BBB.[22] The combined action of these carrier systems results in effective removal of xenobiotics from the CNS, which plays a critical role in drug bioavailability to the brain. The molecular mechanisms involved in the regulation of expression and activity of xenobiotic efflux transporters at the BBB are not fully understood, but proinflammatory cytokines and ROS, both of which are highly relevant to the pathophysiology of TBI, seem to play an important role in this regulation. The data on this aspect of BBB function in traumatized brain are currently not available. It has recently been demonstrated, however, that brain injury resulting from focal cerebral ischemia is associated with a significant upregulation of expression of multidrug resistance 1 (P-glycoprotein) in the cerebrovascular endothelium.[23] P-glycoprotein is an important xenobiotic efflux transporter that can effectively reduce the brain levels of neuroprotective drugs. Pharmacological inhibition of activity of P-glycoprotein or its genetic ablation has been associated with a significant increase in efficacy of neuroprotective interventions in a rodent model of cerebral ischemia.[23] These observations indicate that the therapeutic targeting of xenobiotic efflux transporters at the BBB to restore their normal function after injury may pave the way for more effective neuroprotective treatments. Several single nucleotide polymorphisms have been identified in the multidrug resistance 1 gene in humans, which can affect the biological activity of this transporter. This suggests that the personalized medicine approach may be needed to overcome the hurdles associated with neuroprotective therapies in TBI.

THE ROLE OF NEUROINFLAMMATION IN PATHOPHYSIOLOGY OF TBI

Neuroinflammation plays an important pathophysiological role in TBI. Considerable experimental and clinical data have shown that TBI causes a rapid and substantial increase in CNS synthesis of proinflammatory cytokines, such as tumor necrosis factor α and interleukin 1β. Within hours after the injury, there is a surge in production of these proinflammatory cytokines in the injured brain parenchyma. Proinflammatory cytokines not only promote acute and delayed neuronal death but can also interfere with the survival signals produced by growth factors. In addition, inflammation may have a detrimental effect on neurogenesis occurring after injury. Although the role of proinflammatory cytokines in neuronal repair and long-term recovery is not completely understood, an early anti-inflammatory intervention has demonstrated beneficial therapeutic effects in animal models of TBI. Even in neurotrauma cases where the predominant pathology involves diffuse brain injury that is uncomplicated by contusion, the long-lasting microglial/macrophage activation may take place.[24] These observations underscore the importance of further translational research into this area.

Oxidative Stress and Neuroinflammation

Oxidative stress plays a central role in promoting neuronal death after TBI. ROS are generated through several different cellular pathways, including the calcium-mediated activation of phospholipases, nitric oxide synthase, xanthine oxidase, and the Fenton and Haber-Weiss reactions. The increased production of ROS leads to dysfunction of the BBB. Not only do ROS cause disruption of the BBB, which may result in the formation of posttraumatic vasogenic edema, but also they induce endothelial expression of cell adhesion molecules, promoting invasion of inflammatory cells. ROS also augment the synthesis of many diffusible factors, including a variety of proinflammatory mediators and MMPs. Similar to ROS, the proinflammatory cytokines exert various adverse effects on BBB function, including the disruption of tight junctions and increase in permeability and the induction of expression of cell adhesion molecules. Because ROS induce the production of proinflammatory cytokines and these cytokines have the ability to augment the synthesis of ROS, these two pathophysiological factors may act synergistically through a positive feedback loop.

Posttraumatic Invasion of Inflammatory Cells

Dysfunction of the BBB is central to the progression of neuroinflammation occurring after injury. Brain endothelium itself can be an important source of proinflammatory mediators, such as neutrophil and monocyte chemoattractants. These chemokines are also produced by astrocytes (**Fig. 3**), which participate in generating the chemokine gradients within the injured brain parenchyma and thus facilitate the influx and subsequent movement of inflammatory cells. Increased production of chemokines and augmented expression of cell adhesion molecules on the surface of cerebrovascular endothelium promote invasion of inflammatory cells with detrimental consequences to the integrity of neural tissue. Neutrophils have been known to exacerbate the formation of posttraumatic brain edema[25] and more recent studies have demonstrated that these inflammatory cells are also highly toxic to vulnerable neurons.[26] Similarly, invading monocytes can significantly contribute to the formation of edema and loss of neural tissue in the injured brain.[27,28] Accordingly, treatments directed to counter neutrophil and monocyte influx to the injured brain have shown beneficial therapeutic effects.

The Role of the Choroid Plexus in Brain Inflammatory Response to Injury

Choroid plexus, which is located in all four cerebral ventricles, is a major producer of CSF and together with the arachnoid membrane forms the blood-CSF barrier.

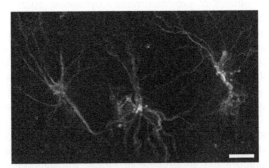

Fig. 3. A confocal microscopy microphotograph showing a cluster of astrocytes in the injured brain parenchyma producing CCL2, a CC chemokine with monocyte chemoattractant properties (bright spots within the soma of astrocytic cells). This immunohistochemical analysis was performed in a rat model of TBI at 6 hours after the insult. Astrocytes were identified using an astrocyte-specific marker, glial fibrillary acidic protein. Astrocytes participate in generating the chemokine gradients within the injured brain parenchyma and thus facilitate the influx and subsequent movement of inflammatory cells. Scale bar = 10 μm.

Although the choroid plexus is usually not directly injured in TBI, recent reports have shown that, in addition to the BBB, it may play an important role in brain inflammatory response to injury.[29,30] The choroid plexus epithelium has the ability to rapidly synthesize and secrete neutrophil chemoattractants in response to injury, and the electron microscopy studies suggest that neutrophils migrate across the choroidal epithelial barrier into the CSF. In a rodent model of TBI, neutrophils have been found to accumulate in the cistern of the velum interpositum, a part of the third cerebral ventricle, and in the subarachnoid CSF space near the injury site, from where these inflammatory cells seemed to migrate to traumatized brain parenchyma.[29] These findings suggest that not only the BBB but also the blood-CSF barrier and CSF-filled space are involved in neutrophil invasion observed after TBI.

BIOMARKERS FOR TBI

The diagnosis and the assessment of neurological injury and outcome of TBI patients are currently based on clinical examination of the level of consciousness using the Glasgow Coma Scale; various imaging techniques, including CT, MRI, and positron emission tomography; and assessment of other vital parameters (eg, ICP and electroencephalogram). These diagnostic tools have been found frustratingly limited, however, prompting the efforts to identify surrogate markers detectable in serum and/or CSF that would provide the information about the extent of neuronal damage resulting from injury and aid in prognosis of outcome. Because CSF samples are frequently not available, particularly from patients with mild to moderate TBI, it is desirable to identify protein biomarkers in serum that are specific for brain tissue and whose levels could be reliably measured. These CNS-derived proteins end up in the peripheral circulation through the process of continual reabsorption of CSF but may also enter the bloodstream through a leaky BBB. Because of a large volume of plasma and the extracellular fluid in peripheral organs, these proteins become substantially diluted, which makes it difficult to measure their serum concentrations. Earlier studies have reported the brain injury–dependent increase in various candidate serum protein markers, such as brain-type creatine kinase, glial fibrillary acidic protein, myelin basic protein, and neuron-specific enolase. Among potential biomarkers that attracted considerable attention is the S100B protein. This protein belongs to a large family of low-molecular-weight (9–13 kDa) S100 proteins with calcium-binding properties. It is most abundant in the cytoplasm of astrocytes and Schwann cells but is also expressed in melanocytes, adipocytes, and chondrocytes, albeit at much lower levels. Although in several studies, S100B has been demonstrated to correlate positively with the severity of injury and negatively with outcome, the recent critical analysis[31] of the validity of S100B as a potential biomarker for TBI has indicated that the serum levels of S100B correlate rather poorly with the levels of this protein in brain tissue and that they primarily depend on the integrity of the BBB, which would be difficult to routinely assess in TBI patients. In addition, the concern has arisen that this marker might not be sufficiently specific for CNS injury. Serum S100B levels have also been shown to increase in response to trauma without head injury or in disorders unrelated to TBI.

With a rapidly growing amount of data on potential protein biomarkers for TBI, it has become increasingly clear that, with the complexity of secondary injury and various time courses of pathophysiological processes involved, it would not be a single protein marker, but, rather, a panel of proteins that could provide useful diagnostic information. Encouraging results have recently been reported from clinical studies where highly sensitive and specific sandwich immunoassays were used to identify a panel of neuron-enriched serum and CSF protein markers for TBI, such as a calpain-derived N-terminal fragment of α-spectrin and phosphorylated forms of neu-rofilament H.[32] Some studies on serum protein biomarkers for TBI using the high throughput proteomic approach involving mass spectrometry techniques have also been conducted.[33,34] These preliminary data require further careful verification by other groups, however, and with the use of other laboratory techniques.

Although major efforts have been directed to identify serum protein markers for TBI, recent studies suggest that plasma microRNAs (miRNAs) may also represent an important class of biomarkers for neurotrauma. miRNAs are small noncoding RNAs that have been shown to possess a considerable level of tissue specificity and suffi-cient stability in plasma. Promising results on plasma miRNA markers have been obtained in animal studies of various forms/models of brain injury and they compared favorably with the data on injuries to peripheral organs,[35,36] suggesting the potential application of these new class of markers for diagnosis and the prediction of outcome in TBI.

PHYSIOLOGICAL ALTERATIONS IN TBI
CBF and Its Autoregulation

The molecular changes induced by TBI, along with dysfunction of the BBB and, in more general terms, the neurovascular unit, can lead to impairments in cerebral vascular and CSF regulation. The brain requires an uninterrupted, generous supply of oxygen and glucose to remain functional, and unlike other organs, does not have high-energy reserves. The brain makes up approximately 2% of body weight but receives 15% to 20% of total cardiac output. The flow and distribution of this high volume of blood, solutes, and nutrients to brain tissues is tightly controlled by homeo-static mechanisms. The remarkable preservation of CBF across a wide range of cere-bral perfusion pressures (CPPs) is called cerebral autoregulation.[37] Autoregulation of CBF is achieved by constant modulation of cerebral vascular resistance and is depen-dent on an intact and functional BBB. CPP is the difference between mean arterial pressure and ICP. When autoregulation of CBF is intact, cerebral arteries respond to a fall in CPP by dilating and maintaining relatively constant perfusion to brain tissue. Although the optimal level for CPP after TBI has been debated, it is generally accepted that CPP below 50 mm Hg is associated with brain tissue ischemia and failure of cere-bral autoregulation. When this happens, CBF and oxygen delivery can fall to levels that cannot sustain normal aerobic metabolism. Although the brain can compensate for decreased CBF by increasing oxygen extraction, this has finite limits. Therefore, very low CPP, which can be caused by low mean arterial pressure, high ICP, or a combination of these changes, carries with it a substantial risk for cerebral ischemia. As discussed previously, ischemia triggers an array of harmful pathophysiological processes, which threaten the structure and function of neurons, glia, and the neuro-vascular unit.[38–41]

The Brain Trauma Foundation Guidelines for the Management of Severe Traumatic Brain Injury and Prognosis recommend that CPP be maintained over 60 mm Hg in patients with severe TBI.[42] Because hypotension (MAP below 90 mm Hg) and hypoxia are seen in more than a third of severe TBI patients, attention to adequate resuscita-tion of blood pressure is a key component of early management of TBI.[43] Clinical investigations have found that 90% of patients who die from TBI have ischemic path-ological changes in the brain, and it is generally agreed that low CPP, BBB dysfunc-tion, and low CBF are key insults that can have a deleterious effect on outcome after TBI.[42] It is difficult to obtain CBF measurements in the early postinjury period in severe TBI. Investigators who have done this have found a correlation between low CBF and more profound neurological deficits and/or mortality.[44,45] In some severe TBI patients, CBF may remain below normal levels for up to 24 hours after injury.[45–48] The majority of TBI patients, however, do not have low CBF or failure of global cerebral autoregulation of CBF. Increasing evidence suggests that alteration of the BBB and failure of autoregulation on a regional or local tissue level may occur without changes in global CBF and may be important in less severe types of TBI, such as concussion.[49] In some TBI patients, especially children, a paradoxical increase in CBF may be seen. This is called luxury perfusion and is thought to be due to loss of autoregulation on the upper end of CPP.

The longer-term recovery of the sensorimotor and higher cortical functions after TBI depends, to a large extent, on adequate blood supply to the brain. A few clinical studies have shown that the reduction in CBF observed in the acute stage may persist for long periods of time after injury.[46–48] In addition, it has been demonstrated that the extent of posttraumatic hypoperfusion is related to the severity of injury and that functional recovery correlates with improvement of CPP. Prolonged (4-week post-TBI) reduction in CBF has also been observed in a rat model of TBI.[49] This post-traumatic hypoperfusion may not be permanent, however, as indicated by recent studies conducted 1 year after trauma in a similar TBI model.[50] These findings suggest that the posttraumatic reduction in CBF may be potentially reversible and that therapeutic interventions aimed at restoring normal blood flow may facilitate functional recovery.

Although cerebral ischemia from low CBF is a threat in the postinjury period, ischemia from vasospasm of cerebral arteries can also occur in the days after severe TBI. Vasospasm has been understood to be a significant part of the pathophysiology of SAH and, with newer imaging and monitoring techniques, is now recognized to also be a factor in TBI. Cerebral vasospasm can lead to ischemic insults and full strokes in patients with severe TBI.[51,52]

Edema and Elevated ICP

The pathologic elevation of ICP is associated with poor outcomes from TBI.[53,54] ICP is normally maintained in adult humans at approximately 7 to 15 mm Hg.[11] Sustained increases in ICP above 20 mm Hg are potentially harmful to the brain due to lower CPP and tissue ischemia. ICP can become elevated in the early postinjury period due to an increase in cerebral blood volume or due to edema. As discussed previously, cytotoxic edema, rather than vasogenic edema, is most likely to result from TBI in humans, but both types can elevate ICP.[11,14]

Therapies targeted at reducing brain edema by osmotic action have been studied in the clinical realm, and mannitol is a recommended treatment for the control of high ICP after TBI. Hypertonic saline has also been investigated but as yet has not shown proved benefit in TBI in large, randomized trials. Although hypertonic saline can reduce brain water content and theoretically reduce edema and ICP, it is not always effective and there is evidence that it can have adverse effects on endothelial cells.[55,56] Better understanding of the pathophysiology of TBI as it relates to ventilation, $PaCO_2$, and CBF has lead to a reversal in the recommendation for hyperventilation as a means controlling high ICP in TBI. Although hyperventilation to a $PaCO_2$ level of less than 35 torr can reduce elevated ICP, it is now understood that prolonged hyperventilation to this level induces cerebral artery vasospasm and reduced CBF to vulnerable brain tissue. Large clinical studies have found that prehospital endotracheal intubation of patients with TBI is associated with increased mortality and worse neurological outcome, and the mechanism for this is most likely inadvertent hyperventilation after intubation.[42,55,57,58]

Pathological Effects of Hemorrhage in TBI

Hemorrhage is another contributing factor to the pathophysiology of TBI and can occur from blunt injury to the skull and brain or penetrating injury. It can also result from secondary injuries, such as cytotoxic edema, ischemia, or intracranial hypertension, when the damaged endothelium of brain capillaries can no longer prevent the extravasation of blood into brain tissues, the subarachnoid space, or the ventricles. Hemorrhage can be minor, and almost incidental, as in the petechial hemorrhages in cortical contusions, or profound and acutely pathological, as in large epidural hematomas that can rapidly expand and cause brain herniation and death. Subdural hemorrhage produces subdural hematomas—one of the most common forms of hemorrhage in TBI. Subdural hematoma is a particular problem in elderly patients who suffer TBI from falls, especially in those patients who are anticoagulated. Hemorrhage may also occur directly into brain tissue as intraparenchymal hemorrhage or into the subarachnoid space as SAH. When SAH occurs in patients with TBI, the same secondary processes that are harmful in aneurismal SAH can occur. In particular, SAH-associated cerebral vasospasm can cause brain ischemia and strokes in the later postinjury period. All brain hemorrhages have the potential to increase ICP by increasing cerebral blood volume.

Apart from its effect on ICP, extravascular blood can participate in many pathological processes. As a rich source of iron, hemoglobin can catalyze the formation of ROS. Blood and hemoglobin can exacerbate secondary injury by stimulating the release of excitatory amino acids and nitric oxide.[59–63] Going beyond red blood cell effects, blood also contains white blood cells and platelets. As discussed previously, white blood cells, especially neutrophils and monocytes, play an important role in brain inflammatory response to injury. Intravascular platelets can cause thrombi in the microcirculation of the brain after TBI.[64]

SUMMARY

The physical forces that cause TBI can directly cause brain tissue destruction and alteration of function. Understanding the biomechanics of TBI, with the unique structure of the skull and the viscoelastic properties of the brain, can help elucidate brain tissue injury zones and patterns.

A complex set of molecular and functional reactions is set in motion by the primary forces in TBI, and the pathological effects of these processes are dependent on the magnitude of the initial injury forces. Whether or not the clinical diagnosis is concussion or severe TBI, however, similar processes are responsible for observed brain dysfunction. The focus on neurons in past research on TBI has perhaps led to an underestimation of the role of the BBB in the dynamic postinjury period. The BBB seems to play a central role in the intrinsic response to injury, and the integrity of the BBB is a major determinant of how pathological processes unfold. AVP may also be an underappreciated part of pathological molecular reactions to TBI, which adversely affect the function of the BBB and promote inflammation. As the response from the initial injury plays out, neuroinflammation is increasingly recognized as a significant part of the equation that determines whether or not a damaging versus healing environment occurs in brain tissue. The prevalence of molecular derangements in TBI holds promise for the identification and use of biomarkers of injury and dysfunction that may be used to assess severity of injury, determine prognosis, or perhaps direct therapy.

The physiological changes in TBI that manifest from the molecular and functional changes at a cellular and tissue level can be measured and modulated. CBF may be reduced globally or only in specific regions of the brain in response to injury. A critical level of CPP—greater than 60 mm Hg—is necessary to keep the brain functioning well after TBI. Elevated ICP is associated with worse outcome after TBI. ICP is affected by many components of the microscopic and macroscopic response to injury, including cellular edema, disruption of the BBB, inflammation, hemorrhage, and production of CSF.

The chronicle of understanding the pathophysiology of TBI provides many examples of how both basic science and clinical investigation have translated into improved management of TBI. In terms of drugs and other therapy, research suggests that a single highly effective pharmacological agent for TBI is unlikely to be discovered but that improved knowledge of the pathophysiology will provide the mechanistic clues to direct a mosaic of therapeutic interventions.

REFERENCES

1. Langlois J, Rutland-Brown W, Wald M. The epidemiology and impact of traumatic brain injury: a brief overview. J Head Trauma Rehabil 2006;21:375–8.
2. Rutland-Brown W, Langlois J, Thomas K, et al. Incidence of traumatic brain injury in the United States, 2003. J Head Trauma Rehabil 2006;21(6):544–8.
3. Jennett B, Teasdale G, Galbraith S. Severe head injury in three countries. J Neurol Neurosurg Psychiatry 1977;40:291–5.
4. Tolias C, Bullock M. Critical appraisal of neuroprotection trials in head injury: what have we learned? NeuroRx 2004;1:71–9.
5. Margulies S, Hicks R. Combination therapies for traumatic brain injury. J Neurotrauma 2009;26:925–39.
6. McLean A. Brain injury without head impact? In: Bandak A, Eppinger R, Ommaya A, editors. Traumatic brain injury: bioscience and mechanics. Larchmont (NY): Mary Ann Liebert, Inc; 1996.
7. Teasdale G, Mathew P. Mechanisms of cerebral concussion, contusion, and other effects of head injury. In: Youmans JR, editor. Neurological surgery. 4th edition. New York: WB Saunders; 1996.
8. Blumbergs P, Scott G, Manavis J, et al. Staining of amyloid precursor to study axonal damage in mild head injury. Lancet 1994;344:1055–6.
9. Thibault L, Gennarelli T. Brain injury: an analysis of neural and neurovascular trauma in the nonhuman primate. Paper presented at: 34th annual proceedings of the Association for the Advancement of Automotive Medicine 1990; Des Plaines (IL).
10. Willinger R, Taleb L, Kopp C. Modal and temporal analysis of head mathematical models. In: Bandak A, Eppinger R, Ommaya A, editors. Traumatic brain injury: bioscience and mechanics. Larchmont (NY): Mary Ann Liebert, Inc; 1996.
11. Smith M. Monitoring intracranial pressure in traumatic brain injury. Anesth Analg 2008;106(1):240–8.
12. Abbott N, Ronnback L, Hansson E. Astrocyte-endothelial interactions at the blood-brain barrier. Nat Rev Neurosci 2006;7:41–53.
13. Baskaya M, Rao A, Dogan A, et al. The biphasic opening of the blood-brain barrier in the cortex and hippocampus after traumatic brain injury in rats. Neurosci Lett 1997;226:33–6.
14. Marmarou A, Signoretti S, Fatouros P, et al. Predominance of cellular edema in traumatic brain swelling in patients with severe head injuries. J Neurosurg 2006;104(5):720–30.

15. Nakayama Y, Takano Y, Shimohigashi Y, et al. Pharmacological characterization of a novel AVP (4–9) binding site in a rat hippocampus. Brain Res 2000;858: 416–23.

16. Szmydynget-Chodobska J, Chung I, Kozniewska E, et al. Increased expression of vasopressin V1a receptors after traumatic brain injury. J Neurotrauma 2004; 21:1090–102.

17. Buijs R, Swaab D, Dogterom J, et al. Intra- and extrahypothalamic vasopressin and oxytocin pathways in the rat. Cell Tissue Res 1978;186:423–33.

18. Chodobski A, Loh Y, Corsetti S, et al. The presence of arginine vasopressin and its mRNA in rat choroid plexus epithelium. Brain Res Mol Brain Res 1997;48: 67–72.

19. Shuaib A, Xu Wang C, Yang T, et al. Effects of nonpeptide V1 vasopression receptor antagonist SR-49059 on infarction volume and recovery of function in a focal embolic stroke model. Stroke 2002;33:3033–7.

20. Trabold R, Kreig S, Scholler K, et al. Role of vasopressin V1a and V2 receptors for the development of secondary brain damage after traumatic brain injury in mice. J Neurotrauma 2008;25:1459–65.

21. Lo E, Singhal A, Torchilin V, et al. Drug delivery to damaged brain. Brain Res Rev 2001;38:140–8.

22. Loscher W, Potschka H. Role of drug efflux transporters in the brain for drug disposition and treatment of brain diseases. Prog Neurobiol 2005;76: 22–76.

23. Spudich A, Kilic E, Xing H, et al. Inhibition of multdrug resistance transporter-1 facilitates neuroprotective therapies after focul cerebral ischemia. Nat Neurosci 2006;2006:487–8.

24. Kelley B, Lifshitz J, Povlishock J. Neuroinflammatory responses after experimental diffuse traumatic brain injury. J Neuropathol Exp Neuroi 2007;66: 989–1001.

25. Schoettle R, Kochanek P, Magargee M. Early polymorphonuclear leukocyte accumlation correlates with the development of post-traumatic cerebral edema in rats. J Neurotrauma 1990;7:207–17.

26. Neumann J, Sauerzweig S, Ronicke R, et al. Microglia cells protect neurons by direct engulfment of invading neutrophil granulocytes: a new mechanism of CNS immune privilege. J Neurosci 2008;28:5965–75.

27. Chen Y, Hallenbeck J, Ruetzler C, et al. Overexpression of monocyte chemoattractant protein 1 in the brain exacerbates ischemic brain injury and is associated with recruitment of inflammatory cells. J Cereb Blood Flow Metab 2003;23: 748–55.

28. Dimitrijevic O, Sm S, Keep R, et al. Absence of the chemokine receptor CCR2 protects against cerebral ischemia/reperfusion injury in mice. Stroke 2007;38: 1345–53.

29. Chodobski A, Chung I, Kozniewska E, et al. Early neutrophilic expression of vascular endothelial growth factor after traumatic brain injury. Neuroscience 2003;122:853–67.

30. Szmydynger-Chodobska J, Strazielle N, Zink B, et al. The role of the choroid plexus in neutrophil invasion after traumatic brain injury. J Cereb Blood Flow Metab 2009;29:1503–16.

31. Kleindienst A, Bullock M. A critical analysis of the role of the neurotrophic protein S100B in acute brain injury. J Neurotrauma 2006;23:1185–200.

32. Siman R, Toraskar N, Dang A, et al. A panel of neuron -enriched proteins as markers for traumatic brain injury in humans. J Neurotrauma 2009;26:1867–77.

33. Haqqani A, Hutchison J, Ward R, et al. Biomarkers and diagnosis; protein biomarkers in serum of pediatric patients with severe traumatic brain injury indentified by ICAT-LC-MS/MS. J Neurotrauma 2007;24:54–74.
34. Hergenroeder G, Redell J, Moore A, et al. Identification of serum biomarkers in brain-injured adults: potential for predicting elevated intracranial pressure. J Neurotrauma 2008;25:79–93.
35. Laterza O, Lim L, Garrett-Engele P, et al. Plasma MircoRNAs as sensitive and specific biomarkers of tissue injury. Clin Chem 2009;55:1977–83.
36. Liu D, Tian Y, Ander B, et al. Brain and blood microRNA expression profiling of ischemic stroke, intracerebral hemorrhage, and kainate seizures. J Cereb Blood Flow Metab 2010;30:92–101.
37. Rangel CL, Gasco J, Nauta H, et al. Cerebral pressure autoregulation in traumatic brain injury. Neurosurg Focus 2008;25(4):E7.
38. Chaiwat O, Sharma D, Udomphorn Y, et al. Cerebral hemodynamic predictors of poor 6-month Glasgow outcome score in severe pediatric traumatic brain injury. J Neurotrauma 2009;26(5):657–63.
39. Figaji A, Zwane E, Fieggan A, et al. Pressure autoregulation, intracranial pressure, and brain tissue oxygentation in children with severe traumatic brain injury. J Neurosurg Pediatr 2009;4(5):420–8.
40. Schmidt B, Klingelhofer J, Perkes I, et al. Cerebral autoregulatory response depends on the direction of change in perfusion pressure. J Neurotrauma 2009;26(5):651–6.
41. Puppo C, Lopez L, Caragna E, et al. One-minute dynamic cerebral autoregulation in severe head injury patients and its comparison with static autoregulation. A transcranial Doppler study. Neurocrit Care 2008;8(3):344–52.
42. Brain Trauma Foundation, American Association of Neurological Surgeons, Congress of Neurological Surgeons, et al. Guidelines for the management and prognosis of severe traumatic brain injury. J Neurotrauma 2007;(24 Suppl 1).
43. Chestnut R, Marshall L, Klauber M, et al. The role of secondary brain injury in determining outcome from severe head injury. J Trauma 1993;34:216–22.
44. Soustiel J, Glenn T, Shik V, et al. Monitoring of cerebral blood flow and metabolism in traumatic brain injury. J Neurotrauma 2005;22(9):955–65.
45. Tisdall M, Smith M. Multimodal monitoring in traumatic brain injury: current status and future directions. Br J Anaesth 2007;99(1):61–7.
46. Obrist W, Langfitt T, ter Weeme C, et al. Non-invasive, long-term, serial studies of rCBF in acute head injury. Acta Neurol Scand Suppl 1977;64:178–9.
47. Obrist W, Gennarelli T, et al. Relation of cerebral blood flow to neurological status and outcome in head-injured patients. J Neurosurg 1979;51:292–300.
48. Jaggi J, Obrist W, Gennarelli T, et al. Relationship of early cerebral blood flow and metabolism to outcome in acute head injury. J Neurosurg 1990;72:176–82.
49. Scremin O, Li M, Scremin A. Cortical contusion induces trans-hemispheric reorganization of blood flow maps. Brain Res 2007;1141:235–41.
50. Kochanek P, Hendrich K, Dixon C, et al. Cerebral blood flow at one year after controlled cortical impact in rats: assessment by magnetic resonance imaging. J Neurotrauma 2002;19:1029–37.
51. Rafols J, Kreipke C, Petrov T. Alterations in cerebral cortex microvessels and the microcirculation in a rat model of traumatic brain injury: a correlative EM and laser Doppler flowmetry study. Neurol Res 2007;29(4):339–47.
52. Oertel M, Boscardin W, Obrist W, et al. Post traumatic vasospasm: the epidemiology, severity, and time course of an underestimated phenomenon: a prospective study performed in 299 patients. J Neurosurg 2005;103(5):812–24.

53. Carter B, Butt W, Taylor A. ICP and CPP excellent predictors of long term outcome in severely brain injured children. Childs Nerv Syst 2008;24(2):245–51.
54. Lin J, Tsai J, Lin C, et al. Evaluation of optimal cerebral perfusion pressure in severe traumatic brain injury. Acta Neurochir Suppl 2008;101:131–6.
55. Soustiel J, Mahamid E, Chistyakov A, et al. Comparison of moderate hyperventilation and mannitol for control of intracranial pressure control in patients with severe traumatic brain injury—a study of cerebral blood flow and metabolism. Acta Neurochir (Wien) 2006;148(8):845–51.
56. Cooper D, Myles P, McDermott F. Prehospital hypertonic saline resuscitation of patients with hypotension severe traumatic brain injury: a randomized controlled trial. JAMA 2004;291(11):1350–7.
57. Wang H, Cassidy L, Adelson P, et al. Out of hospital endotracheal intubation and outcome after traumatic brain injury. Ann Emerg Med 2004;44:439–50.
58. Stiell I, Nesbitt L, Pickell W, et al. The OPALS major trauma study: impact of advanced life support on survival and morbidity. CMAJ 2008;178(9):1141–52.
59. Perez de la Ossa N, Sobrino T, Silva Y. Iron-related brain damage in patients with intracerebral hemorrhage. Stroke 2010;2010(41):4.
60. Schnuriger B, Inaba K, Abdelsayed G, et al. The impact of platelets on the progression of traumatic intracranial hemorrhage. J Trauma 2010;68(4):881–5.
61. Strbian D, Kovanen P, Karjalainen-Lindsberg M, et al. An emerging role of mast cells in cerebral ischemia and hemorrhage. Ann Med 2009;1:1–13.
62. Yilmazlar S, Hanci M, Oz B, et al. Blood degradation products play a role in cerebral ischemia caused by acute subdural hematoma. J Neurosurg Sci 1997;41: 379–85.
63. Regan R, Panter S. Hemoglobin potentiates excitotoxic injury in cortical cell culture. J Neurotrauma 1996;13(4):223–31.
64. Schwarzmaier S, Kim S, Trabold R, et al. Temporal profile of thrombogenesis in the cerebral microcirculation after traumatic brain injury in mice. J Neurotrauma 2010;27(1):121–30.

Blast-induced Mild Traumatic Brain Injury

Gregory A. Elder, MD[a,b,c,]*, Effie M. Mitsis, PhD[b,d],
Stephen T. Ahlers, PhD[e], Adrian Cristian, MD[d,f]

KEYWORDS

- Blast-related brain injury • Improvised explosive device
- Posttraumatic stress disorder • Traumatic brain injury

Traumatic brain injury (TBI) has been a major cause of mortality and morbidity in the wars in Iraq and Afghanistan, known as Operation Iraqi Freedom (OIF) and Operation Enduring Freedom (OEF). In the popular press, TBI has sometimes been referred to as the signature injury of the Iraq and Afghanistan wars,[1] with estimates that 10% to 20% of returning OIF/OEF veterans have suffered a TBI.[2–6] Most attention focused initially on moderate to severe TBIs recognized in theater,[7] and OIF has resulted in the highest number of service-related severe TBIs since the Vietnam era.[8]

However, it soon became apparent that many OIF/OEF veterans were presenting to Veteran's Affairs (VA) hospitals and other facilities with symptoms suggestive of the residual effects of mild TBIs that were never recognized before discharge. Mild TBIs greatly outnumber moderate to severe TBIs in this population.[2,3] Although diverse mechanisms have resulted in injury, because of the prominent use of improvised

Work in the author's labs is supported by grants from the Department of Veterans Affairs (1I01RX000179-01 and I01CX000190-01). The views expressed in this article are those of the authors and do not necessarily reflect the official policy or position of the Department of the Navy, Department of Defense, or the United States Government.

[a] Neurology Service, James J. Peters Department of Veterans Affairs Medical Center, 130 West Kingsbridge Road, Bronx, NY 10468, USA

[b] Department of Psychiatry, Mount Sinai School of Medicine, One Gustave L. Levy Place, New York, NY 10029, USA

[c] Department of Neurology, Mount Sinai School of Medicine, One Gustave L. Levy Place, New York, NY 10029, USA

[d] Rehabilitation Medicine Service, James J. Peters Veterans Affairs Medical Center, 130 West Kingsbridge Road, Bronx, NY 10468, USA

[e] Operational and Undersea Medicine Directorate, Naval Medical Research Center, 503 Robert Grant Avenue, Silver Spring, MD 20910, USA

[f] Department of Rehabilitation Medicine, Mount Sinai School of Medicine, One Gustave L. Levy Place, New York, NY 10029, USA

* Corresponding author. Neurology Service, James J. Peters Veterans Affairs Medical Center, 130 West Kingsbridge Road, Bronx, NY 10468.
E-mail address: gregory.elder@va.gov

Psychiatr Clin N Am 33 (2010) 757–781
doi:10.1016/j.psc.2010.08.001
0193-953X/10/$ – see front matter. Published by Elsevier Inc.

psych.theclinics.com

explosive devices (IEDs) in both theaters of operation, blast exposure has been the most common cause of TBI.[2-5] More broadly, according to Department of Defense (DoD) statistics of February 6 2010, of the more than 41,000 US military casualties in Iraq and Afghanistan, more than 26,000 were caused by explosive devices.[9] There are concerns that blast-related TBIs may produce both long-term health effects in veterans as well as affecting the in-theater performance of active-duty troops.

This review discusses some of the current controversies related to mild TBI, in particular the distinction between mild TBI and posttraumatic stress disorder (PTSD). The problem of distinguishing between the 2 disorders is not new and has roots dating back to the historical entity known as shell shock.[10] During World War I (WWI), while British troops were engaged in the static trench warfare that was characteristic of fighting on the frontlines in Europe, they were exposed to a variety of blasts at close range, including artillery barrages and mortar attacks. In this era before the advent of steel helmets, symptoms developed that were reminiscent of both the post-concussion syndrome and what would now be called PTSD. A variety of names for this entity were used but the most enduring label was shell shock. The disorder became so common during WWI that 10% of British battle casualties were diagnosed with shell shock, accounting for one-seventh of all discharges from the British Army, one-third of cases when physical wounds were excluded. A vigorous debate took place concerning whether shell shock represented a physical injury or was the result of psychic trauma. The debate ended without any clear resolution, but with most clinicians probably favoring a psychological explanation. As World War II (WWII) began, hoping to avoid another epidemic, including associated pension claims, the British government went so far as to ban the use of the term shell shock.[10] Despite this, soldiers continued to be exposed to blasts and to present with a similar range of symptoms. The controversy regarding physical versus psychological injury continued without any clear resolution.

MECHANISMS OF BLAST-RELATED INJURY

A variety of explosives including mortar shells, rocket propelled grenades, and IEDs cause blast injuries. In Iraq and Afghanistan, IEDs have been the most common cause of blast injuries and are estimated to be responsible for about 40% of coalition deaths in Iraq, and a roughly similar percentage of TBIs.[11] Although diverse in design, IEDs typically consist of an explosive charge coupled to a detonator.[12] The explosive charge may be a conventional artillery shell or be made from commercially manufactured or homemade explosives. IEDs often incorporate shrapnel-generating materials including nails, ball bearings, scrap metal, or other particulate material. Devices used to trigger IEDs may be sophisticated or simple, ranging from electronic transmitters to trip wires, tilt switches, motion detectors, or thermal or pressure-sensitive switches. IEDs are often placed along transport routes and triggered to detonate beneath vehicles. Vehicle-borne devices may contain large quantities of explosives and are placed in strategic locations or driven into their targets.

During a detonation, a solid or liquid explosive is converted nearly instantaneously into a gas, creating a pulse of increased air pressure lasting only milliseconds.[12-16] The gases rapidly expand as a sphere from the point source, forming a high-pressure wave, known as the blast overpressure wave (**Fig. 1**). The overpressure wave travels faster than the speed of sound and is followed closely by a blast wind generated by the mass displacement of air caused by the expanding gases. Following the overpressure wave, pressure decreases creating a relative vacuum or blast underpressure wave during which a momentary reversal of airflow or reversed blast wind occurs.

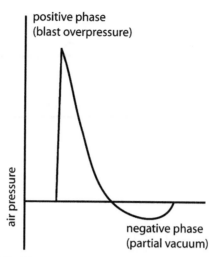

Fig. 1. Components of the blast pressure wave. As gases expand rapidly a high-pressure wave traveling at supersonic speeds is generated (the blast overpressure wave). As pressure decreases, a relative vacuum is created that momentarily leads to a reversal of airflow. A second lower-intensity positive-pressure wave follows before atmospheric pressure returns to normal. See text and Refs.[12–16] for additional discussion.

The underpressure wave is followed by a second positive-pressure wave before atmospheric pressure returns to normal.

Blast injuries occur through multiple mechanisms.[12,13,15] Injuries directly related to the initial blast wave are referred to as primary blast injuries. In addition to primary injuries, the blast wind that follows the overpressure wave can propel objects including shrapnel contained within the IED, causing secondary injury. The blast wave may also cause the individual to be knocked down or thrown into solid objects, resulting in tertiary injury. A group of miscellaneous injuries, including burns or the effects of inhaling noxious gases or other toxic exposures, may also result and are termed quaternary injuries. A type of injury termed a quinary pattern has been suggested to exist, based on a series of 4 cases in Israel in which hyperpyrexia and other autonomic disturbances in association with a hyperinflammatory state was noted following exposure to a bomb blast.[17]

Depending on the type and amount of explosive, the velocity of the blast wave in air may be extremely high. When the blast wave impacts the human body, part of the wave is reflected or deflected but most of the wave is absorbed and propagated through the body.[16,18,19] The result is generation of high-frequency stress waves and lower-frequency shear waves. Stress and shear waves are believed to injure tissues through multiple mechanisms including spallation, implosion, and inertial effects.[12,15,16,18] Spallation results when a pressure wave passes from a medium of greater to lesser density, resulting in displacement and fragmentation of the dense medium into the less dense. For example, an explosive detonated under water forces the denser water to spall into the less dense air, causing fragmentation that is observed as an upward splash. Implosion forces result when gases within tissues are suddenly compressed by the blast overpressure. Tissues may be damaged by collapsing on themselves or, as the positive-pressure wave passes, gases re-expand and release kinetic energy that may damage tissue. Inertial or shearing forces occur when tissues of different densities are propelled at different speeds as the overpressure wave passes through organs or tissues.[12,16,18] These forces are similar in their pathophysiological effects to the acceleration/deceleration forces that occur in closed-impact TBIs, such as those associated with motor vehicle accidents, when tissues of different densities may be damaged by their collision with one another, or the cytoarchitecture of a tissue may be disrupted.

Factors that affect the degree of primary blast injury include distance from the detonation, the blast wave's peak overpressure, its duration, and other characteristics of the overpressure wave form.[15,16,18] The orientation of the body to the blast wave, as well as environmental factors, may also influence primary blast effects. For example, explosions within enclosed structures or adjacent to walls become amplified by shockwave reflection and cause greater injury than if exposure occurs in an open space.[12]

Organs regarded as most vulnerable to blast effects are those having air-fluid interfaces.[12,13] The tympanic membrane is regarded as the most susceptible structure in the body, and ruptured tympanic membranes have been commonly observed in relation to blast injuries in Iraq and Afghanistan.[13,20–22] The lungs and abdominal viscera are also highly sensitive to primary blast injury, with pulmonary injury being one of the most common life-threatening injuries in those close to detonation.[12,13]

THE PRIMARY BLAST WAVE AND THE BRAIN

How the primary blast wave affects the brain is at present incompletely understood. Computer simulations[23–29] predict various potential mechanisms of injury, including induction of high strain effects in traditional coup and contrecoup regions[29] and high shear stresses in white matter regions that could be associated with diffuse axonal injury (DAI).[23] Some models also predict preferential damage to the brainstem.[29] Others suggest that, as the blast wave passes through the head because of the mechanical properties of the skull, there is significant blast pressure magnification caused by reflection of the blast wave off the skull, with the highest mechanical damage predicted in focal areas on the opposite side of the head.[24] Blast waves have also been predicted to generate sufficient force to produce potentially damaging skull flexures.[25]

Besides direct effects of the primary blast wave on brain, a thoracic mechanism has also been proposed to contribute to brain injury.[30,31] Specifically, this theory proposes that a high-pressure blast wave hitting the body compresses the abdomen and chest, inducing oscillating high-pressure waves that can be transmitted through the systemic circulation to the brain, leading to preferential damage to cellular elements close to cerebral vessels. It has also been suggested that blast overpressure may cause sudden hyperinflation of the lungs, inducing a vasovagal response that could lead to apnea, bradycardia, and hypotension, causing cerebral hypoxemia.[15]

Understanding the mechanisms that underlie primary blast injury has practical implications for protection of troops in the field. In particular, the thoracic mechanism implies that even blast-resistant helmets would not protect against brain injury. In addition, although current body armor protects the trunk from projectile injuries, there are suggestions that it may intensify the blast wave by serving as an improved contact surface for shock propagation[31] or serve as a reflecting surface that concentrates the energy of the blast wave by causing it to resonate internally.[15] If the thoracic hypothesis is correct, new types of body armor would need to be designed that could absorb or deflect blast wave energies to prevent central nervous system (CNS) injury.

Other mechanisms of CNS injury that have been suggested include that the primary blast wave may cause formation of air emboli leading to cerebral infarction.[32] It has been also suggested that the blast wave may be focused through the orbital sockets and nasal sinuses, causing preferential injury to the orbitofrontal cortex.[33]

EXPERIMENTAL STUDIES IN ANIMALS

Animals have been exposed to various forms of blast ranging from direct exposure to live explosives to controlled blast waves produced by compressed-air generators. In most studies, to concentrate the blast wave, anesthetized animals have been placed in special holders designed to limit body movement. The animals are secured in the end of a metal tube termed a shock tube if live explosives are used or a blast tube if compressed air is used. Effects of body alignment can be determined by altering the animal's orientation within the tube and, by applying appropriate shielding, it is possible to isolate the effects of body versus head exposure. An example of a blast tube apparatus is shown in **Fig. 2**.

Although live explosives may best model exposure in the field, this approach affords less experimental control over the physical characteristics of the blast wave as well as difficulty in separating primary from secondary injury. Pressure generators allow blast overpressure effects to be studied in isolation, offering more experimental control. However, a limitation of both shock and blast tubes is that, although they replicate the ideal blast wave, they lack the capability to model the nonideal blast wave, with its multiple shock and expansion fronts, that occurs in real-life settings. Some studies have used open-field exposure or exposure in simulated bunkers or other types of enclosures. For example, Bauman and colleagues[34] recently described a swine model of blast injury in which, in addition to exposure in a blast tube, pigs were exposed to an explosive charge detonation while secured in a simulated Humvee or in a 4-sided building.

Several studies have looked at the effect of blast exposure on the CNS **(Table 1)**. Most have used rats but some have studied rabbits,[35] pigs,[34,36,37] or nonhuman primates.[38] One study examined the effects of blast injury to the brain in whales at sea.[39] The choice of species has both practical and theoretical implications. Practically, rodents are less expensive to study than larger animals. However, rodents suffer the disadvantage of having smooth brains lacking the gyri, sulci, and proportion of white matter found in human brain, anatomical factors that may affect the mechanical properties of the brain's reaction to blast exposure. Species such as pigs and nonhuman primates offer the advantage of having a brain more similar to humans, but a significant disadvantage lies in their cost and availability.

Studies in rats and pigs have established that the primary blast wave is transmitted through the skull to the brain.[34,40] In pigs, a transient flattening of the electroencephalogram (EEG) with apnea has been observed immediately after blast exposure[36]; effects that might, in part, be explained by the vasovagal mechanism alluded to earlier. However, disruption of the EEG in pigs has been seen when the head, but not the body, was exposed to blast injury,[34] arguing that a cerebral mechanism may be involved. Prominent vasospasm has also been shown angiographically immediately following blast injury in pigs.[34]

Pathologically, high-level blast exposure seems particularly prone to inducing hemorrhagic lesions including intraparenchymal, subdural, and subarachnoid bleeding. Blast injury also induces a variety of histological effects including neuroaxonal, glial, microglial, and myelin abnormalities, sometimes with apoptotic neurons (see **Table 1**). Increased energy consumption and evidence of oxidative stress have been observed, as well as persistent cognitive and motor deficits.

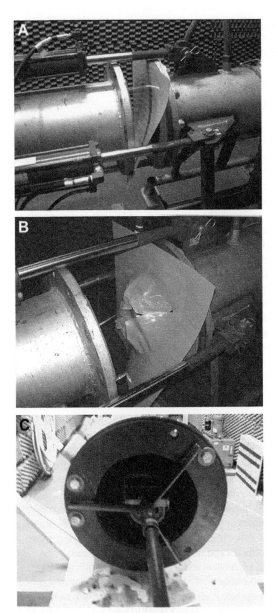

Fig. 2. (A, B, C) An experimental shock tube. The shock tube consists of a horizontally mounted, 30-cm diameter, circular, 4.1-m long, steel tube. The tube is divided into a 0.76-m compression chamber separated from a 5.18-m expansion chamber by 1 or more polyethylene Mylar sheets (Du Pont Co, Wilmington, DE, USA) depending on the peak pressure desired. The shock tube depicted is housed in the Walter Reed Army Institute of Research.

Animal studies have provided mixed support for the thoracic hypothesis,[31] with one study finding higher intrathoracic pressures and increased mortality when sheep exposed to blast were fitted with a cloth ballistic vest,[41] whereas, in other studies,[42] placement of a soft body armor comparable to a Kevlar vest on the thorax and part of the abdomen reduced mortality and ameliorated the widespread fiber degeneration that was prominent in brains of unprotected rats during exposure to a 126-kPa blast. The importance of vagally mediated effects has been supported by experiments in rabbits[55] and rats[43] that found that animals with bilateral vagotomies had less brady-cardia, hypotension, and apnea; effects that could contribute to cerebral damage. Axonal degeneration in the optic nerve and central visual pathways has also been observed,[44] an effect consistent with suggestions that blast forces may be focused by the orbital sockets.[33]

One limitation of most animal studies to date is that they have used relatively powerful blast exposures delivered to anesthetized animals at levels high enough to induce significant pulmonary pathology.[45–47] Only a few studies have examined effects of lower-level blasts that are probably more comparable with the mild TBI exposures that are the most common exposure in the current war zones. Moochhala and colleagues[48] studied the effects of 2.8- to 20-kPa exposures in rats. Although blast-exposed animals showed no deficits in a passive avoidance-learning task, the 20 kPa–exposed animals showed impaired motor function, and histologically scattered hyperchromatic and apoptotic neurons were found in the cerebral cortex 24 hours after exposure. Saljo and colleagues[49] also found that exposure of rats to 10- to 60-kPa blasts increased intracranial pressure in a dose-dependent manner and cognitive function, as judged by a Morris water maze, was impaired at 2 days after exposure to 10- or 30-kPa blasts. Collectively, these studies clearly indicate that the primary blast wave has CNS effects and that these effects may be apparent even at modest blast pressures.

BLAST-RELATED TBI IN HUMANS

Blast injury is infrequent in civilian life. A survey of 57,392 trauma cases seen in a large urban trauma center found only 89 cases of blast injury (0.2%),[50] with private dwelling explosions and industrial accidents being the most common causes. The best under-stood pathophysiological mechanisms associated with the type of blunt impact TBI seen most commonly in civilian settings are bleeding, direct tissue damage, and DAI.[51] DAI results when angular forces cause shearing or stretching of axons that can lead to impaired axonal transport that is pathologically associated with focal axonal swellings. DAI is common following closed head injuries and most commonly affects tracts at gray/white matter junctions, particularly in frontal and temporal regions. Contusions occur as the result of coup/contrecoup injuries, most affecting the frontotemporal regions and occipital lobes.

It is unclear whether blast-related brain injury is similar to the blunt impact injury seen in civilian life or whether blast injury may produce pathophysiologically distinct changes. Few human cases of blast exposure have come to autopsy and all of them sustained such severe injuries that they died within a few days of injury.[52] The most prominent features in 2 cases from WWI studied by Mott[53] were multiple punc-tate hemorrhages in subcortical gray and white matter regions. Cohen and Biskind[54] identified 9 cases from WWII in the archives of the Armed Forces Institute of Pathology, all whom died within 5 days of injury. These cases also exhibited a promi-nent hemorrhagic component with diffuse leptomeningeal bleeding, intracerebral clots, and multifocal hemorrhages in white matter.

Close exposure to a high-pressure blast wave can clearly cause moderate to severe TBI, likely activating many of the same pathophysiological cascades seen in closed impact injury. However, these injuries are a mix of secondary and tertiary injuries, making the contribution of primary blast difficult to ascertain. Belanger and

Table 1
Blast-related CNS effects in animal studies

Species	Blast Exposure	Peak[a] Pressure	CNS Effects	References
Rhesus monkey	Air pressure–driven shock tube	207, 276, and 345 kPa	Transient impairment in performance on auditory and visual discrimination avoidance task	38
Rabbit	Air pressure–driven shock tube	304 kPa	Acutely in medulla oblongata, increased lipid peroxidation products, glucose and lactate concentrations, lactate/pyruvate ratio and increased phosphocreatine/adenosine triphosphate ratio, all indicative of increased energy consumption	35
Rat	Air pressure–driven shock tube	104–110 and 129–173 kPa	Axonal degeneration in the optic nerve and central visual pathways	44
Pig	Open exposure to RDX/TNT mixture	200–300 kPa	Reduction of amplitude of EEG immediately after blast accompanied by apnea	36
Rat	Air pressure–driven shock tube	338.9 kPa	Swollen neurons; glial reaction; myelin debris; increased pinocytotic activity; increased total nitrite/nitrate; increased superoxide dismutase activity, superoxide anion and malondialdehyde generation; decreased glutathione peroxicase activity; impaired performance active avoidance task	45,46
Rat	Nitrate-based conventional explosive (TNT compound B); exposed in a simulated bunker	Equivalent to 110 kg TNT	Transient widespread microglial response in various brain regions and presence of cells expressing major histocompatibility complex class I and II (Ia) antigen and neurons in the cerebral and cerebellar cortex with darkened dendrites; transient disruption of the ultrastructure of the choroid plexus with widened perivascular spaces and the presence of cells expressing immune-related markers among the epiplexus cells	102–104

Rat	Pentaerythrittetranitrate plastic explosive in a metal tube	154 or 240 kPa	Redistribution of phosphorylated neurofilament H protein from axon to perikarya; induction of c-jun, c-fos, c-myc, and β-amyloid precursor protein in neurons in multiple brain regions including hippocampus and cortex; induction of scattered neuronal apoptosis; microglial reaction and induction of GFAP-positive astrocytes	105–108
Minke whale	Harpoon tipped with a grenade containing 30 g penthrite	Unknown	Extensive macroscopic and microscopic intracerebral, subarachnoid and subdural hemorrhage, severity related to proximity of explosion to head	39
Rat	Pentaerythrittetranitrate plastic explosive in a metal tube detonated in concrete bunker	2.8 or 20 kPa	Decreased rotarod and grip strength in 20 kPa–exposed animals; scattered hyperchromatic and TUNEL-positive apoptotic cells in cerebral cortex after 20 kPa exposure; effects of blast reversed by aminoguanidine	48
Rat	Air pressure–driven shock tube	40 kPa	Transmission of blast pressure waves to brain	40
Rat	Single shock produced by silver azide explosion applied directly to the brain after craniotomy	1 or 10 MPa	At 10 MPa, gross and microscopic hemorrhage in cortical and subcortical regions; induction of apoptotic neurons with evidence of caspase 3 activation; at 1 MPa, spindle-shaped changes in neurons and elongation of neuronal nuclei without other evidence of damage	109
Pig	Firing of a howitzer, bazooka, or automatic rifle in open air; automatic rifle fire in concrete enclosure; local body exposure from air pressure–driven shock tube; underwater exposure	9–30 kPa	Blast wave transmitted to brain; at 30-kPa exposure grossly visible subdural, subarachnoid, and intraparenchymal hemorrhages; microscopic intraparenchymal hemorrhages	37
Rat	Air pressure–driven shock tube	126 and 147 kPa	Hemorrhage, necrosis and widespread fiber degeneration in brain; impaired beam walking and impaired spatial learning in Morris water maze; less fiber degeneration in 126 kPa–exposed animals wearing a Kevlar vest	42

(continued on next page)

Table 1
(continued)

Species	Blast Exposure	Peak[a] Pressure	CNS Effects	References
Pig	Binary uncased explosive charge in blast tube, simulated Humvee or building	Variable 62–179 kPa	Angiographically demonstrated vasospasm in brain immediately after blast; EEG flattening during blast exposure; persistent impairment of motor coordination; prominent fiber degeneration and GFAP-positive astroglial reaction; increased myelin basic protein and neuron-specific enolase in serum	34
Rat	Air-driven shock tube, 3 exposures in 20 min	10, 30, and 60 kPa	Increased intracranial pressure after blast returned to normal by 7 d; spatial memory impaired in Morris water maze; effects blocked by feeding a processed cereal feed compared with standard feed	49

Abbreviations: EEG, electroencephalogram; GFAP, glial fibrillary acidic protein; RDX, hexogene; TNT, trinitrotoluene; TUNEL, terminal deoxynucleotidyl transferase-mediated dUTP nick-end labeling.

[a] For consistency, data have been converted to kPa where original blast pressures were given in pounds per square inch (psi).

colleagues[55] compared neuropsychological test results in a group of primarily OIF/ OEF veterans who sustained TBIs as a result of blast versus those who sustained TBIs from blunt force trauma and found no major differences in patterns between blast and non–blast-injured subjects, thus providing no support at the neuropsychological level that blast is different. However, distinct pathophysiological mechanisms might produce similar functional consequences. It is also unclear whether long-term effects may be caused by a primary blast wave sufficient only to produce mild TBI and whether multiple exposures to this type of blast, which is common among troops in Iraq,[2] can lead to significant long-term effects. There are few neuropathological data on mild TBI in general, and none related to blast-induced mild TBI.

NEUROIMAGING IN MILD TBI

Use of in vivo measures to understand the mechanisms of brain damage, particularly mild TBI, as a result of acute and repeated exposure to blast is in its infancy. Conventional structural imaging techniques such as computed tomography (CT) and magnetic resonance imaging (MRI) have been used historically in both civilian and military patients with TBI, and are capable of rapid identification of contusions or hemorrhages in the dural and parenchymal spaces as well as cerebral edema. However, these techniques often result in negative findings in nonblast, civilian mild TBI (data on the use of CT and MRI in military patients following blast exposure is limited at this juncture), because they are considered to be less sensitive to the small size of mild TBI lesions and to DAI,[56,57] which is widely hypothesized to be a principle mechanism of damage in mild TBI. Hence, an absence of visible damage on structural scans does not necessarily mean an absence of abnormality, as the lesions associated with mild TBI may be too small, thus failing to achieve the current threshold of detection for these techniques.[58,59] In addition, conventional MRI is sensitive to blood from torn vessels but is not sensitive to axonal damage itself, thus likely underestimating the presence of DAI, especially in milder cases of injury in which hemorrhagic lesions are uncommon.

Functional imaging, such as positron emission tomography (PET), is also used in the evaluation of TBI but is not typically the standard of practice in clinical or military settings during the acute stage of assessment in mild TBI. PET studies have been used extensively in research studies evaluating brain glucose metabolic activity and cerebral blood flow in civilian patients with TBI and have contributed considerably to understanding of abnormalities in subtle brain injury. Recent studies suggest that PET imaging may be more sensitive to mild trauma than is conventional structural imaging such as CT or MRI.[60,61] For example, PET imaging has often shown abnormalities in mild TBI that show some correlation with prognosis, Glasgow Coma Scale (GCS), and neuropsychological deficits in the absence of findings on structural imaging. In what may be an important direction in the understanding of chronic symptoms of mild TBI in the absence of findings on CT or MRI, and thus for clinical practice, recent review articles[60,61] have generally concluded that functional brain imaging is more sensitive than anatomical imaging in the period of months and even years after the injury.[62]

Diffusion tensor imaging (DTI) is a new imaging technique that provides a more direct measure of the integrity of white matter fibers via the DTI metrics of fractional anisotropy (FA) and mean diffusivity (MD). White matter tracts normally constrain the isotropic diffusion of water. An FA value approaching 1.0 reflects maximal anisotropic diffusion, and values approaching zero indicate compromised white matter integrity. The MD values are typically increased in brain trauma, but may be decreased, depending on TBI severity or the time frame in which DTI is conducted after injury (eg, see Refs.[63–66]). Because DTI is considered to be sensitive to subtle forms of damage and to DAI, it holds promise as a sensitive tool in identifying impairment in blast-related mild TBI.

An increasing number of DTI studies, conducted primarily in civilian mild TBI, have emerged. Most,[56,65,67–69] but not all,[63,64,66] of these studies indicate reductions in FA at sites of axonal shearing injury, indicating reduced directionality in the diffusion of water molecules. The discrepancies found in some of these studies in outcomes (ie, decreased or increased FA) may be related to scanning in the acute versus chronic phase of injury, age of the patient population (adolescent vs adults), methodology used, and selection of regions of interest. Newer studies exploring the relationship between DTI and cognitive outcomes have shown significant correlations between DTI findings and neuropsychological function, particularly in the cognitive domains of learning, memory, and processing speed.[68,70–73]

In response to funding opportunities initiated primarily by the DoD and the Veterans Affairs Administration to address the effects of blast in military personnel, neuroimaging in OIF/OEF veterans with mild TBI is now being conducted by investigators at several VA medical centers across the country. Using more sensitive imaging methods to show brain abnormalities in veterans with chronic postconcussive symptoms years after their last exposure to blast will undoubtedly inform the debate as to whether blast mild TBI is a distinct pathophysiological entity. Identifying biomarkers specific to blast would improve diagnostic accuracy, treatment interventions, and overall patient management.

To our knowledge, only 2 studies have been published with findings in postdeployed veterans and service members with both mild and moderate blast TBI,[74,75] 1 using [^{18}F]fluoro-2-deoxyglucose PET (FDG PET)[75] and the other DTI.[74] Peskind and colleagues[75] compared 12 Iraq war veterans with a mean age of 32 years who had at least 1 blast exposure that resulted in acute mild TBI as defined by the American Congress of Rehabilitation Medicine criteria and had persistent postconcussive symptoms with a group of civilian controls who were, on average, 20 years older than the veteran group. At the time of PET scanning, veterans were on average 3.5 ($\pm$ 1.2) years after their last exposure to blast. Compared with controls, veterans with blast exposure mild TBI with or without PTSD showed consistent regional hypometabolism in infratentorial (cerebellum, vermis, and pons) and medial temporal regions. Veterans also exhibited subtle impairments in complex information processing, some reductions in verbal fluency, processing speed, and aspects of attention and working memory. These findings are the first to show with FDG PET that blast exposure resulting in mild TBI may have a neurobiological substrate that is measurable and that the persistent postconcussive symptoms with which so many OIF/OEF veterans present at VA hospitals should not be solely attributed to psychiatric disorders until the contribution of structural brain injury has been fully evaluated and established.

In the 1 published study using DTI, Levin and colleagues[74] examined the effects of mild to moderate blast-related TBI in 37 OIF/OEF veterans and service members (mean age 31.5 $\pm$ 7.2 years) who were on average 871.5 ($\pm$ 343.1) days after injury compared with a group of OIF/OEF veterans without blast exposure (N = 15) who sustained injury to other body regions or had no injury. Using manual measurement of single-slice regions of interest, quantitative tractography, and voxel-based methods of DTI analysis, this group found no between-group differences in white matter integrity. The distributions of FA and the apparent diffusion coefficient were similar across neuroanatomic regions of white matter known to be vulnerable to axonal injury. The correlations between DTI data and postconcussion symptoms were weak. Definitive conclusions regarding blast exposure mild TBI cannot be determined from the findings of 1 study. The Levin and colleagues[74] study may be especially limited by the sample size of the comparison group, which was less than half of the blast-exposed group Furthermore, there is a lack of information regarding specifics of the comparison group (ie, type of extracranial injuries that were present in 8 of the 15 subjects).

Systematic and comprehensive studies using functional imaging methods in veterans and service members with blast exposure mild TBI with acute and chronic postconcussive symptoms are beginning to emerge. These comprehensive studies are timely because of the significant number of veterans returning from Iraq and Afghanistan with chronic and disabling sequelae of brain injury. Advanced neuroimaging techniques hold promise for the detection and characterization in vivo of subthreshold, but clinically significant, abnormalities in blast mild TBI.

DISTINGUISHING BLAST-RELATED MILD TBI FROM PTSD

One of the striking features of the mild TBI cases being seen in the current OIF/OEF veterans is the high prevalence of PTSD. PTSD or depression is present in more than one-third of OIF/OEF veterans with suspected postconcussion syndromes secondary to mild TBI.[2] This coincidence could reflect dual exposure to blast as well as stressors that can independently cause PTSD. However, the clinical distinction between a postconcussion syndrome and PTSD is often difficult, with the 2 disorders having many overlapping symptoms. In both disorders, complaints of fatigue, irritability, and poor sleep are frequent. Impaired concentration, attention, and memory are also common symptoms and neuropsychological test profiles may look similar with deficits in attention, working memory, executive functioning, and episodic memory prominent in both disorders.[76] In practice, when a documented episode of TBI is present, the clinical distinction between the 2 disorders is usually based on the predominant symptoms, a postconcussion syndrome being suspected when patients have more organic symptoms such as headache, dizziness, visual complaints, hearing loss, balance problems, and cognitive disturbance, whereas PTSD is more likely to be diagnosed when the predominant symptoms include nightmares, hyperarousal, avoidance, and re-experiencing phenomena. The more severe cognitive impairments and associated neurological deficits make cases of moderate to severe TBI easy to recognize. What is more difficult is separating the postconcussion syndrome of mild TBI from PTSD, and sometimes even deciding whether a TBI has occurred may be difficult in cases of mild TBI in which distinguishing transient neurological dysfunction from a psychologically based stress reaction is not always easy.

An increasing number of reports are beginning to address the issue of overlap. The first such study was that of Hoge and colleagues[2] who surveyed more than 2700 US Army infantry soldiers from 2 brigades, 3 to 4 months after returning from a 1-year deployment in Iraq. Questionnaires were used to elicit information regarding the occurrence of a TBI and other injuries during deployment as well as current general health status and the presence of symptoms suggestive of a postconcussion syndrome, PTSD, or depression. The most frequent TBI exposure was blast and, among the sample, 5% reported a TBI with loss of consciousness (LOC) that was most typically on the order of a few seconds to 3 minutes. Ten percent reported a TBI without LOC (ie, reported being dazed/confused), giving a total of 15% reporting a TBI. All but 4 of the 384 TBIs reported were mild TBIs. In soldiers who reported a mild TBI, complaints of headache and poor memory and concentration were frequent, suggesting that a persistent postconcussion syndrome was present. Of those reporting

TBI with LOC, 44% met criteria for PTSD, whereas PTSD was present in 27% of those reporting altered mental status without LOC. In addition, major depression was present in 23% and 8% respectively. This high coincidence of PTSD and depression led the investigators to perform a covariate analysis for the 2 disorders and, after adjusting for the coexistence of PTSD and depression, a mild TBI history was no longer significantly associated with adverse physical health outcomes or symptoms, except for headache.

In a subsequent study, this same group determined whether a blast mechanism identifies individuals at higher risk of persistent postconcussive symptoms following TBI.[5] Anonymous surveys were administered to 3952 US Army infantry soldiers 3 to 6 months after returning from a year-long deployment to Iraq; 14.9% of the total sample met criteria for having suffered a concussion with most (72.2%) reporting a blast mechanism of injury. Of those who suffered a concussion, 34.2% reported LOC and 63.5% only an alteration of consciousness. Among those with LOC, a blast mechanism was associated with headaches and tinnitus. However, among soldiers reporting only transient alterations of consciousness without LOC, blast was not associated with adverse health outcomes, arguing that a history of blast exposure was associated with persistent postconcussive symptoms only in those whose TBI involved LOC and not most mild TBI cases as currently defined.

In a large randomly selected cohort of more than 5800 UK military personnel deployed to Iraq, Fear and colleagues[77] also found that postconcussive symptoms were associated with exposure to blast during deployment. However, similar symptoms were as likely to occur with other in-theater experiences not associated with blast exposure, such as aiding the wounded or potential exposure to depleted uranium. They concluded that postconcussive symptoms are common in returning troops and, although some may be related to blast exposure, the association is not specific.

One interpretation of these findings is that the current screening procedures and definitions of mild TBI are flawed[78] and that much of what is presently being called blast-related mild TBI is really PTSD. Similar suggestions have been made concerning the postconcussion syndrome following closed head injuries in civilian cases, with one prospective study reporting that postconcussive symptoms are as common following trauma without TBI as with mild TBI.[79] Clearly, many of the symptoms of postconcussion syndrome overlap with PTSD and are not specific to either disorder.

However, other studies have suggested that the link may be more than coincidental. Mora and colleagues[80] reviewed the records of 333 patients admitted consecutively to the United States Army Institute of Surgical Research burn center for explosion-related injuries between March 2003 and March 2006 and examined the prevalence of PTSD in patients with burns with and without primary blast injury or mild TBI as defined by LOC. They found a greater prevalence of PTSD in patients with burns with primary blast injury and mild TBI than in patients with burns injured by other mechanisms. Walilko and colleagues,[81] in a study of 124 survivors of the Oklahoma City bombing, explored the relationships between PTSD and physical injuries. They found a significant association between PTSD and head/brain injuries, whereas PTSD was not highly correlated with other injuries. Collectively, these studies could be seen as arguing that TBI may predispose to the development of PTSD.

TBI and PTSD can be considered as different ends of a spectrum, with TBI being the classic example of an organic brain disease and PTSD a psychologically based reaction to a stressor that was not associated with physical injury. Indeed, it has been suggested that the posttraumatic amnesia associated with TBI may protect against PTSD, based on the notion that amnesia for the event precludes formation of the core affective responses associated with the development of PTSD.[82] There are likely mitigating factors that allow the development of PTSD even in the context of amnesia for the event, including that, in the context of mild TBI, amnesia may be only partial, allowing for some aspects of the experience to be encoded.[83] In addition, secondary sources such as family or friends may provide enough information to allow the victim to reconstruct the incident, and experiences in the posttrauma period, such as events witnessed after regaining consciousness or subsequent medical procedures, may be psychologically traumatic in and of themselves. PTSD has been documented in moderate and severe TBI.[83] However, one prospective study found that PTSD rates were higher in subjects who remembered the TBI incident compared with those with no memory for the event.[84] Studies on whether PTSD rates are higher in mild compared with moderate or severe TBI have given more mixed results.[83,85] Stress experiences are also typically not limited to single, isolated events, and service personnel in a war zone inevitably have exposure to PTSD stressors independent of TBI events, making coexistence of the 2 disorders easy to imagine.

A second possibility to explain the PTSD/TBI interface is that the 2 conditions are not coincidental but rather that TBI may increase the risk of developing PTSD following a psychological trauma. Physical injury of any type, even if not involving the brain, has been reported to increase the risk of developing PTSD.[86] Studies of Vietnam veterans have also suggested that TBI is associated with more severe PTSD[87] and, in OEF/OIF veterans, PTSD is more prevalent in veterans reporting mild TBI, compared both with veterans who suffered no injury[2,6] or with those who suffered injuries not involving the head.[2] In the study by Hoge and colleagues,[2] mild TBI was associated with PTSD even after controlling for the intensity of combat experience.

These observations thus raise the question of whether a neural insult might alter reactions to psychological stressors and increase the likelihood that PTSD will develop. One mechanism whereby TBI might predispose to PTSD would be if blast-related injury damaged brain structures that are involved in the development of PTSD.[33,76,88,89] Current biological models of PTSD postulate that key frontal and limbic structures, including the prefrontal cortex, amygdala, and hippocampus, are involved in the development of PTSD.[76,90,91] These models suggest that a key component of the disorder is inadequate frontal inhibition of the amygdala, a limbic structure believed to be central to the fear response and the formation of fear associations. Exaggerated amygdala responses are believed to heighten responses to psychological threats. A substantial body of functional neuroimaging data is consistent with such models, suggesting that there is heightened amygdala activity with decreased hippocampal and orbital frontal activity in PTSD,[90,91] and, in a study of penetrating brain injuries in Vietnam veterans, damage to the amygdala was associated with less PTSD compared with other lesion locations.[92] Damage to the prefrontal cortex by TBI could therefore predispose individuals to abnormally sustained responses to psychological stressors. Damage to regions such as the hippocampus might also impair the cognitive reserve needed to deal with psychological stressors afterward.

At present, the regional specificity of blast-related brain injury is not known. What is also not known is the degree to which subclinical blast exposure (ie, not sufficient to produce a transient neurological alteration qualifying as a TBI) may affect the brain. Multiple subclinical exposures are common in the war zones in Iraq and Afghanistan and could affect the brain even in the absence of a diagnosable TBI event. Largely because of research in the sport's medicine literature, the definition of concussion, which used to require LOC, has been expanded to include even the most transient alterations of consciousness. If subclinical blast exposure affects the brain, this definition would need to be expanded even further to capture the full spectrum of blast effects on brain, and would suggest that the TBI model may be misleading with regard to blast and fail to capture what is really a spectrum of blast-related brain injury.

The distinction between blast-related brain injury and PTSD has more than academic significance because it affects treatment strategies as well as patient education. The pathophysiology of PTSD is most commonly conceptualized as an abnormally sustained stress response. Treatment of PTSD is focused on normalization of stress reactions through psychologically based as well as pharmacologically based treatments, the latter often involving the use of selective serotonin reuptake inhibitors. By contrast, TBI treatments are based on an organic model that presumes that structural brain alterations have occurred and that recovery depends on neurological factors. Treatments focus on improving attention and concentration with agents such as psychostimulants, or improving compensatory strategies through cognitive-behavioral therapies. Pharmacological interventions that improve one condition may worsen the other.[90] For example, α-adrenergic blockers such as prazosin, which are given to improve sleep in PTSD, may worsen TBI-related cognitive complaints, and agents that improve cognitive function, such as methylphenidate, may exacerbate PTSD symptoms. It is also possible that persistent cognitive deficits associated with TBI may complicate cognitive-behavioral approaches to PTSD because both exposure-based and cognitive-behavioral interventions depend on some measure of cognitive reserve, making it plausible that cognitive deficits associated with TBI may reduce responsiveness to PTSD therapies.

The diagnosis of TBI may also be viewed as carrying the implication of permanent brain injury, and labels can unintentionally affect prognosis. By contrast, although the diagnosis of PTSD may be regarded as more benign in one sense, it still carries a stigma in the minds of some. This attitude may be particularly prevalent in the culture of the military, in which service personnel may be more comfortable and receptive of treatment depending on the diagnosis.

DIAGNOSIS AND SCREENING FOR BLAST-RELATED TBI

The diagnosis of moderate to severe TBI is straightforward even in theater because the traumatic incident is generally apparent along with prolonged alterations of consciousness; other clinical signs and symptoms, and often neuroimaging abnormalities, are discovered later. By contrast, accurate identification of mild TBI can be challenging because of the more subtle signs of injury, the paucity of objective physical findings, and the overlap of postconcussion symptoms with those of other disorders including depression, PTSD, and the effects of chronic pain. In theater, it can even be difficult to establish whether a TBI event has occurred because of the transient nature of the neurological dysfunction and the difficulty of distinguishing TBI from an acute stress reaction. The problem is compounded by the diagnosis frequently not being made until much later when it is difficult for the veteran to recall the events surrounding a blast that occurred several months or even years earlier. It is often difficult to reconstruct the time course of the veteran's present symptoms in relation to the TBI event, information that is critical to establishing the existence of a postconcussion syndrome. Soldiers in these wars are also in constant exposure to blasts, some close by and some at a distance, and the effects of repeated subclinical exposure to blasts (ie, less than the threshold of producing a TBI event) are unknown.

It is important to obtain as many details about specific events as possible. Good detective work is often necessary. Obtaining medical records or talking to key people familiar with the event can be challenging, but it can yield useful information. As in civilian head trauma, the diagnosis of blast-related mild TBI is largely based on establishing an accurate history of the specific events that led to a brain injury. It is important to determine whether there was direct trauma to the brain (ie, falls, motor vehicle accidents, bullets) or indirect trauma (ie, close exposure to blasts). It is clearly important to establish the presence of symptoms such as headaches, dizziness, impaired balance, memory loss, inability to focus, difficulty making decisions, mental fatigue, irritability, and problems with sleep soon after the event and their persistence to the present day. In addition, the effects of these symptoms on current functioning and interpersonal relationships should be ascertained: For example, are they having difficulties at work keeping up with job requirements or getting along with supervisors and coworkers? If in school, are they receiving low grades in course work? To what extent have the often-reported behavioral changes (irritability, low frustration tolerance, anger outbursts) affected their lives? The effect of these symptoms on key social relationships with spouses, children, and friends should also be determined.

The physical examination is often limited in aiding the diagnosis of mild TBI in blast-injured veterans, especially if they are far removed from the immediate event. Nevertheless, a thorough neurological and cognitive examination should be performed that assesses orientation, concentration, immediate and delayed recall, as well as motor strength, balance, and gait. Assessment for tympanic membrane rupture is also important because this has been described as a marker of concussive blast injury in soldiers.[13,20–22] Standard neuroimaging, such as CT scan and MRI, are often not helpful, but should be considered on a case-by-case basis. Current research is exploring the usefulness of functional imaging as an adjuvant to the diagnostic process. One new technique being used in blast-related mild TBI is DTI, which holds promise as a sensitive tool in identifying impairment in mild injury (as discussed earlier). Although there is much interest in establishing biomarkers for TBI,[94,95] none currently exist.

To deal with the problem of missed cases, both the DoD and VA have implemented population-based screening procedures for mild TBI.[3,96,97] In recognition of the importance of early diagnosis, the DoD in 2007 implemented screening processes throughout the course of combat operations, beginning with troops in the field who may have experienced a blast-related TBI. As soon as practical, soldiers are evaluated by medics using a structured assessment tool, the Military Acute Concussion Evaluation (MACE).[98] The MACE consists of 13 items (8 history and 5 examination). In the history assessment, the clinician records details of the incident. Items such as a description of the event, cause of the injury (ie, explosion, blast, fall, motor vehicle accident, gunshot wound), wearing of a helmet, amnesia surrounding the event, LOC, and symptoms are recorded. In the examination, the clinician evaluates 5 domains: (1) orientation; (2) immediate memory; (3) neurological screening of vision, speech, and motor function; (4) concentration; and (5) delayed recall. Total maximum score for the examination is 30. Scores less than 25 may indicate cognitive impairment.[98] The usefulness of this instrument for predicting subsequent functional impairment has not been established, but it holds the potential for providing the most objective history regarding the initial injury.

More recently, for screening in the field, the DoD has moved away from what has been called a symptom-based approach to an incident-based approach to facilitate early detection.[99] This new protocol, which was being implemented in spring 2010, makes medical evaluations mandatory for those involved in incidents such as being close to explosions or blasts, whereas, in the past, evaluations were performed after such incidents only if soldiers reported symptoms. As part of this initiative, the DoD is also focusing on educating commanders as well as troops in the field on the symptoms of TBI and the importance of early diagnosis and treatment.

Service members returning from OIF/OEF undergo a range of mandatory health assessments as part of their Postdeployment Health Assessment, which includes assessment for self-reported TBIs. One of these assessments, the Brief Traumatic Brain Injury Screen (BTBIS) comprises 3 questions designed to determine whether an injury occurred, whether that injury was associated with a TBI, and whether there are current symptoms that are consistent with an ongoing postconcussion syndrome.[96] The BTBIS is used to identify those who may have sustained an injury that was not identified acutely. Since May 2008, baseline neurocognitive testing before deployment has been performed using the Automated Neuropsychological Assessment Metrics (ANAM)[97]. The ANAM TBI military battery is completed during a 15-minute computerized assessment and includes tests of code substitution, simple reaction time, matching to sample, reaction time, and mathematical processing. The ANAM thus provides a baseline against which cognitive functioning after injury can be compared.

The VA has mandated TBI screening for all OIF/OEF veterans who present to VA hospitals for any reason, using a 4-question screening procedure,[96] the basis of which is, like the BTBIS, to establish whether a TBI event is likely to have occurred and whether the veteran is currently symptomatic. Although such screens lack specificity and are subject to both false-positive and false-negative results, they are suitable for large-scale postdeployment screening.[96] The VA has also established a polytrauma/TBI system of care nationwide to deal with identified cases.[100] A positive screen triggers referral to a clinic within this network where a secondary TBI evaluation is performed. If a TBI is confirmed, the veteran is referred for appropriate clinical services.

Research efforts are also underway, both within the VA and DoD, to increase understanding of the pathophysiology and natural history of blast-related TBI.[97] Among these efforts are the establishment of a DoD TBI registry and studies to validate the MACE as well as other screening tools. Active efforts are also underway to apply the most modern neuroimaging techniques to blast-related TBI and to use advanced computer modeling methods to simulate the effects of blast.

TREATMENT PRINCIPLES FOR THE VETERAN WITH A BLAST-RELATED MILD TBI

The cornerstones in the treatment of veterans with mild TBI are education, symptom management, and care coordination. Veterans and their families are educated on the causes, symptoms, treatments, and prognosis of mild TBI. The educational interventions take into account the veteran's cognitive and emotional impairments as well as their cultural and religious beliefs and preferred method of learning. Educational materials must be written at an appropriate reading level and in a language that the veteran can readily understand. The information provided often needs to be repeated at several visits and by different providers, therefore consistency in the content and method of education by all providers is important.

In educating the veteran with a mild TBI, it is important that the instruction occurs in a quiet environment that is conducive to learning and that an adequate amount of time is allowed for the visits. Material can be reinforced through alternate means such as telephone calls whenever necessary. Family education is critical to the successful reintegration of the veteran back to the community and home life. Families are encouraged to participate in educational activities and support groups. Some examples of general educational content include (1) compensatory strategies for impaired memory and concentration; (2) relaxation techniques; (3) anger management techniques; (4) diet and exercise; (5) strategies for successful reintegration in work, school, and social activities; (6) limiting alcohol and caffeine intake; and (7) avoidance of high-risk behavior that could increase the risk of additional head injuries.

The symptoms associated with mild TBI can be broadly divided into 3 groups: physical, cognitive, and behavioral. It is common for veterans to complain of concurrent symptoms in each of these groups. It is therefore important to prioritize and treat the symptoms that cause the veteran the most distress first. Although the treatment of specific symptoms associated with mild TBI is beyond the scope of this article, some general principles are briefly discussed. The reader is directed to the VA/DoD Clinical Practice Guideline for more specific treatment recommendations in this population.[101]

Injured brains are sensitive to the side effects of medications, therefore close monitoring during treatment is suggested to evaluate for potential toxicities and drug-drug interactions. Clinicians should avoid medications that can lower the seizure threshold, cause drowsiness or slow thinking, as well as those medications associated with increasing risk of suicidal ideation, because suicide risk is higher in this population.

Some commonly used interventions in the symptom management of veterans with mild TBI include (1) physical therapy for the treatment of musculoskeletal pain syndromes and balance disorders; (2) voice recorders, global positioning systems (GPS) and personal digital assistants as aids to veterans with memory impairments; (3) cognitive remediation training; (4) sunglasses for veterans whose eyes are sensitive to sunlight; (5) speech pathology referrals for teaching of communication skills; (6) mental health referrals for management of depression, PTSD, and anxiety; (7) referrals to substance abuse treatment specialists as needed; (8) teaching of sleep management techniques such as avoidance of alcohol, avoidance of caffeine products, stimulants, and nicotine before a sleep period, waking up at regular times, avoidance of naps during the daytime, and stimulating activities immediately before sleep. Vigilance for conditions such as sleep apnea is recommended, with referrals for sleep studies or to sleep specialists as needed.

Case management in this population is important to ensure that care is coordinated and that social service needs are adequately addressed. The veteran should also be educated on return to activities such as work, school, and leisure. The decision on when and how to return is made based on the severity of the cognitive, physical, and emotional impairments and the type of work previously engaged in. Safety is a primary consideration if the veteran previously engaged in high-risk work. Another consideration is the ability to perform specific tasks with competence. Successful reintegration may involve a period of work restriction or accommodation such as provision of additional time to complete tasks and working in a quiet environment with additional supervision.

CONCLUDING REMARKS

TBI has been a major cause of mortality and morbidity in the wars in Iraq and Afghanistan. In both theaters of operation, blast exposure has been the most common cause of TBI. Blast injuries occur through multiple mechanisms that likely activate many of the same pathophysiological cascades seen in closed impact injuries in civilian life. What is less clear is whether the primary blast wave causes brain damage through mechanisms that are pathophysiologically distinct from those common in civilian TBI and, in particular, whether multiple exposures to low-level blast can lead to long-term sequelae. One of the other striking features of the mild TBI cases being encountered in OIF/OEF veterans is the high prevalence of PTSD. At present, it is unclear whether this association reflects coincident exposure or whether the relationship is more complex with, for example, TBI increasing the risk of developing PTSD by damaging brain structures that are involved in mediating PTSD. Resolution of these issues affects treatment strategies as well as strategies for protection of troops in the field and is an area of high priority for research both within the DoD and Department of Veteran's Affairs.

REFERENCES

1. Alvarez L. War veterans' concussions are often overlooked. New York Times. August 25, 2008: A1.
2. Hoge CW, McGurk D, Thomas JL, et al. Mild traumatic brain injury in U.S. soldiers returning from Iraq. N Engl J Med 2008;358:453–63.
3. Tanielian T, Jaycox LH, editors. Invisible wounds of war: psychological and cognitive injuries, their consequences, and services to assist recovery. Santa Monica (CA): Rand Corporation; 2008.
4. Terrio H, Brenner LA, Ivins BJ, et al. Traumatic brain injury screening: preliminary findings in a US Army Brigade Combat Team. J Head Trauma Rehabil 2009,24.14–23.
5. Wilk JE, Thomas JL, McGurk DM, et al. Mild traumatic brain injury (concussion) during combat: lack of association of blast mechanism with persistent postconcussive symptoms. J Head Trauma Rehabil 2010;25:9–14.
6. Schneiderman AI, Braver ER, Kang HK. Understanding sequelae of injury mechanisms and mild traumatic brain injury incurred during the conflicts in Iraq and Afghanistan: persistent postconcussive symptoms and posttraumatic stress disorder. Am J Epidemiol 2008;167:1446–52.
7. Warden DL, Ryan L, Helmick K, et al. War neurotrauma: the defense and veterans brain injury center (DVBIC) experience at the Walter Reed Army Medical Center. J Neurotrauma 2005;22:1178.
8. Bell RS, Vo AH, Neal CJ, et al. Military traumatic brain and spinal column injury: a 5-year study of the impact blast and other military grade weaponry on the central nervous system. J Trauma 2009;66:S104–11.
9. Available at: http://siadapp.dmdc.osd.mil/personnel/CASUALTY/castop.htm. Accessed February 6, 2010.
10. Jones E, Fear NT, Wessely S. Shell shock and mild traumatic brain injury: a historical review. Am J Psychiatry 2007;164:1641–5.
11. Brookings Institution, Saban Center for Middle East Policy. Iraq index: tracking variables of reconstruction and security in post-Saddam Iraq. April 27, 2010. Available at: www.brookings.edu/iraqindex. Accessed May 2, 2010.
12. Wolf SJ, Bebarta VS, Bonnett CJ, et al. Blast injuries. Lancet 2009;374:405–15.
13. DePalma RG, Burris DG, Champion HR, et al. Blast injuries. N Engl J Med 2005; 352:1335–42.
14. Taber KH, Warden DL, Hurley RA. Blast-related traumatic brain injury: what is known? J Neuropsychiatry Clin Neurosci 2006;18:141–5.
15. Cernak I, Noble-Haeusslein LJ. Traumatic brain injury: an overview of pathobiology with emphasis on military populations. J Cereb Blood Flow Metab 2010; 30:255–66.
16. Leung LY, VandeVord PJ, Dal Cengio AL, et al. Blast related neurotrauma: a review of cellular injury. Mol Cell Biomech 2008;5:155–68.
17. Kluger Y, Nimrod A, Biderman P, et al. The quinary pattern of blast injury. Am J Disaster Med 2007;2:21–5.
18. Clemedson CJ. Blast injury. Physiol Rev 1956;36:336–54.
19. Howe LL. Giving context to post-deployment post-concussive-like symptoms: blast-related potential mild traumatic brain injury and comorbidities. Clin Neuropsychol 2009;23:1315–37.
20. Okie S. Traumatic brain injury in the war zone. N Engl J Med 2005;352:2043–7.

21. Xydakis MS, Bebarta VS, Harrison CD, et al. Tympanic-membrane perforation as a marker of concussive brain injury in Iraq. N Engl J Med 2007;357:830–1.

22. Ritenour AE, Wickley A, Ritenour JS, et al. Tympanic membrane perforation and hearing loss from blast overpressure in Operation Enduring Freedom and Operation Iraqi Freedom wounded. J Trauma 2008;64:S174–8.

23. Chafi MS, Karami G, Ziejewski M. Biomechanical assessment of brain dynamic responses due to blast pressure waves. Ann Biomed Eng 2009;38:490–504.

24. Moore DF, Jerusalem A, Nyein M, et al. Computational biology - modeling of primary blast effects on the central nervous system. Neuroimage 2009;47 (Suppl 2):T10–20.

25. Moss WC, King MJ, Blackman EG. Skull flexure from blast waves: a mechanism for brain injury with implications for helmet design. Phys Rev Lett 2009;103: 108702.

26. Taylor PA, Ford CC. Simulation of blast-induced early-time intracranial wave physics leading to traumatic brain injury. J Biomech Eng 2009;131: 061007.

27. Zhang J, Pintar FA, Yoganandan N, et al. Experimental study of blast-induced traumatic brain injury using a physical head model. Stapp Car Crash J 2009; 53:215–27.

28. Zhang J, Song B, Pintar FA, et al. How to test brain and brain simulant at ballistic and blast strain rates. Biomed Sci Instrum 2008;44:129–34.

29. Zhang J, Yoganandan N, Pintar FA, et al. A finite element study of blast traumatic brain injury - biomed 2009. Biomed Sci Instrum 2009;45:119–24.

30. Bhattacharjee Y. Neuroscience. Shell shock revisited: solving the puzzle of blast trauma. Science 2008;319:406–8.

31. Courtney AC, Courtney MW. A thoracic mechanism of mild traumatic brain injury due to blast pressure waves. Med Hypotheses 2009;72:76–83.

32. Phillips YY, Richardson D. Primary blast injury: a brief history. In: Zatchuck R, Jenkins D, Bellamy R, et al, editors. Textbook of military medicine. Part I. Warfare, weapons and the casualty, Conventional warfare. Ballistic, blast and burn injuries, vol. 5. Washington DC: TMM Publications; 1990. p. 221–40.

33. Hoffman SW, Harrison C. The interaction between psychological health and traumatic brain injury: a neuroscience perspective. Clin Neuropsychol 2009;23: 1400–15.

34. Bauman RA, Ling G, Tong L, et al. An introductory characterization of a combat-casualty-care relevant swine model of closed head injury resulting from exposure to explosive blast. J Neurotrauma 2009;26:841–60.

35. Cernak I, Savic J, Malicevic Z, et al. Involvement of the central nervous system in the general response to pulmonary blast injury. J Trauma 1996;40:S100–4.

36. Axelsson H, Hjelmqvist H, Medin A, et al. Physiological changes in pigs exposed to a blast wave from a detonating high-explosive charge. Mil Med 2000;165:119–26.

37. Saljo A, Arrhen F, Bolouri H, et al. Neuropathology and pressure in the pig brain resulting from low-impulse noise exposure. J Neurotrauma 2008;25: 1397–406.

38. Bogo V, Hutton R, Bruner A. The effects of airblast on discriminated avoidance behavior in rhesus monkeys. In: Technical progress report on contract no. DA-49-146-XZ-372, vol. DASA 2659. Washington, DC: Defense Nuclear Agency; 1971. p. 1–32.

39. Knudsen SK, Oen EO. Blast-induced neurotrauma in whales. Neurosci Res 2003;46:377–86.

40. Chavko M, Koller WA, Prusaczyk WK, et al. Measurement of blast wave by a miniature fiber optic pressure transducer in the rat brain. J Neurosci Methods 2007;159:277–81.

41. Phillips YY, Mundie TG, Yelverton JT, et al. Cloth ballistic vest alters response to blast. J Trauma 1988;28:S149–52.

42. Long JB, Bentley TL, Wessner KA, et al. Blast overpressure in rats: recreating a battlefield injury in the laboratory. J Neurotrauma 2009;26:827–40.

43. Irwin RJ, Lerner MR, Bealer JF, et al. Shock after blast wave injury is caused by a vagally mediated reflex. J Trauma 1999;47:105–10.

44. Petras JM, Bauman RA, Elsayed NM. Visual system degeneration induced by blast overpressure. Toxicology 1997;121:41–9.

45. Cernak I, Wang Z, Jiang J, et al. Cognitive deficits following blast injury-induced neurotrauma: possible involvement of nitric oxide. Brain Inj 2001;15:593–612.

46. Cernak I, Wang Z, Jiang J, et al. Ultrastructural and functional characteristics of blast injury-induced neurotrauma. J Trauma 2001;50:695–706.

47. Chavko M, Prusaczyk WK, McCarron RM. Lung injury and recovery after exposure to blast overpressure. J Trauma 2006;61:933–42.

48. Moochhala SM, Md S, Lu J, et al. Neuroprotective role of aminoguanidine in behavioral changes after blast injury. J Trauma 2004;56:393–403.

49. Saljo A, Bolouri H, Mayorga M, et al. Low-level blast raises intracranial pressure and impairs cognitive function in rats: prophylaxis with processed cereal feed. J Neurotrauma 2010;27:383–9.

50. Bochicchio GV, Lumpkins K, O'Connor J, et al. Blast injury in a civilian trauma setting is associated with a delay in diagnosis of traumatic brain injury. Am Surg 2008;74:267–70.

51. Gennarelli TA, Grahm DI. Neuropathology. In: Silver JM, McAllister TW, Yudofsky SC, editors. Textbook of traumatic brain injury. Arlington (VA): American Psychiatric Publishing; 2005. p. 27–50.

52. Kocsis JD, Tessler A. Pathology of blast-related brain injury. J Rehabil Res Dev 2009;46:667–72.

53. Mott F. The effects of high explosives upon the central nervous system. Lancet 1916;1:441–9.

54. Cohen H, Biskind G. Pathologic aspects of atmospheric blast injuries in man. Arch Pathol 1946;42:12–34.

55. Belanger HG, Kretzmer T, Yoash-Gantz R, et al. Cognitive sequelae of blast-related versus other mechanisms of brain trauma. J Int Neuropsychol Soc 2009;15:1–8.

56. Arfanakis K, Haughton VM, Carew JD, et al. Diffusion tensor MR imaging in diffuse axonal injury. AJNR Am J Neuroradiol 2002;23:794–802.

57. Huisman TA, Schwamm LH, Schaefer PW, et al. Diffusion tensor imaging as potential biomarker of white matter injury in diffuse axonal injury. AJNR Am J Neuroradiol 2004;25:370–6.

58. Bigler ED. Quantitative magnetic resonance imaging in traumatic brain injury. J Head Trauma Rehabil 2001;16:117–34.

59. Bigler ED, Snyder JL. Neuropsychological outcome and quantitative neuroimaging in mild head injury. Arch Clin Neuropsychol 1995;10:159–74.

60. Newberg AB, Alavi A. Neuroimaging in patients with head injury. Semin Nucl Med 2003;33:136–47.

61. Van Heertum RL, Greenstein EA, Tikofsky RS. 2-Deoxy-fluorglucose-positron emission tomography imaging of the brain: current clinical applications with emphasis on the dementias. Semin Nucl Med 2004;34:300–12.

62. Kato T, Nakayama N, Yasokawa Y, et al. Statistical image analysis of cerebral glucose metabolism in patients with cognitive impairment following diffuse traumatic brain injury. J Neurotrauma 2007;24:919–26.
63. Bazarian JJ, Zhong J, Blyth B, et al. Diffusion tensor imaging detects clinically important axonal damage after mild traumatic brain injury: a pilot study. J Neurotrauma 2007;24:1447–59.
64. Chu Z, Wilde EA, Hunter JV, et al. Voxel-based analysis of diffusion tensor imaging in mild traumatic brain injury in adolescents. AJNR Am J Neuroradiol 2010;31:340–6.
65. Inglese M, Makani S, Johnson G, et al. Diffuse axonal injury in mild traumatic brain injury: a diffusion tensor imaging study. J Neurosurg 2005;103:298–303.
66. Wilde EA, McCauley SR, Hunter JV, et al. Diffusion tensor imaging of acute mild traumatic brain injury in adolescents. Neurology 2008;70:948–55.
67. Kraus MF, Susmaras T, Caughlin BP, et al. White matter integrity and cognition in chronic traumatic brain injury: a diffusion tensor imaging study. Brain 2007;130:2508–19.
68. Lipton ML, Gellella E, Lo C, et al. Multifocal white matter ultrastructural abnormalities in mild traumatic brain injury with cognitive disability: a voxel-wise analysis of diffusion tensor imaging. J Neurotrauma 2008;25:1335–42.
69. Miles L, Grossman RI, Johnson G, et al. Short-term DTI predictors of cognitive dysfunction in mild traumatic brain injury. Brain Inj 2008;22:115–22.
70. Levin HS, Wilde EA, Chu Z, et al. Diffusion tensor imaging in relation to cognitive and functional outcome of traumatic brain injury in children. J Head Trauma Rehabil 2008;23:197–208.
71. Mathias JL, Bigler ED, Jones NR, et al. Neuropsychological and information processing performance and its relationship to white matter changes following moderate and severe traumatic brain injury: a preliminary study. Appl Neuropsychol 2004;11:134–52.
72. Niogi SN, Mukherjee P, Ghajar J, et al. Extent of microstructural white matter injury in postconcussive syndrome correlates with impaired cognitive reaction time: a 3T diffusion tensor imaging study of mild traumatic brain injury. AJNR Am J Neuroradiol 2008;29:967–73.
73. Salmond CH, Menon DK, Chatfield DA, et al. Diffusion tensor imaging in chronic head injury survivors: correlations with learning and memory indices. Neuroimage 2006;29:117–24.
74. Levin HS, Wilde E, Troyanskaya M, et al. Diffusion tensor imaging of mild to moderate blast-related traumatic brain injury and its sequelae. J Neurotrauma 2010;27:683–94.
75. Peskind ER, Petrie EC, Cross DJ, et al. Cerebrocerebellar hypometabolism associated with repetitive blast exposure mild traumatic brain injury in 12 Iraq war Veterans with persistent post-concussive symptoms. Neuroimage [Epub ahead of print]. PMID: 20385245.
76. Vasterling JJ, Verfaellie M, Sullivan KD. Mild traumatic brain injury and posttraumatic stress disorder in returning veterans: perspectives from cognitive neuroscience. Clin Psychol Rev 2009;29:674–84.
77. Fear NT, Jones E, Groom M, et al. Symptoms of post-concussional syndrome are non-specifically related to mild traumatic brain injury in UK Armed Forces personnel on return from deployment in Iraq: an analysis of self-reported data. Psychol Med 2009;39:1379–87.
78. Hoge CW, Goldberg HM, Castro CA. Care of war veterans with mild traumatic brain injury–flawed perspectives. N Engl J Med 2009;360:1588–91.

79. Meares S, Shores EA, Taylor AJ, et al. Mild traumatic brain injury does not predict acute postconcussion syndrome. J Neurol Neurosurg Psychiatry 2008;79:300–6.

80. Mora AG, Ritenour AE, Wade CE, et al. Posttraumatic stress disorder in combat casualties with burns sustaining primary blast and concussive injuries. J Trauma 2009;66:S178–85.

81. Walilko T, North C, Young LA, et al. Head injury as a PTSD predictor among Oklahoma City bombing survivors. J Trauma 2009;67:1311–9.

82. Joseph S, Masterson J. Posttraumatic stress disorder and traumatic brain injury: are they mutually exclusive? J Trauma Stress 1999;12:437–53.

83. Harvey AG, Brewin CR, Jones C, et al. Coexistence of posttraumatic stress disorder and traumatic brain injury: towards a resolution of the paradox. J Int Neuropsychol Soc 2003;9:663–76.

84. Gil S, Caspi Y, Ben-Ari IZ, et al. Does memory of a traumatic event increase the risk for posttraumatic stress disorder in patients with traumatic brain injury? A prospective study. Am J Psychiatry 2005;162:963–9.

85. Glaesser J, Neuner F, Lutgehetmann R, et al. Posttraumatic stress disorder in patients with traumatic brain injury. BMC Psychiatry 2004;4:5.

86. Koren D, Norman D, Cohen A, et al. Increased PTSD risk with combat-related injury: a matched comparison study of injured and uninjured soldiers experiencing the same combat events. Am J Psychiatry 2005;162:276–82.

87. Vanderploeg RD, Belanger HG, Curtiss G. Mild traumatic brain injury and posttraumatic stress disorder and their associations with health symptoms. Arch Phys Med Rehabil 2009;90:1084–93.

88. Bryant RA. Disentangling mild traumatic brain injury and stress reactions. N Engl J Med 2008;358:525–7.

89. Elder GA, Cristian A. Blast-related mild traumatic brain injury: mechanisms of injury and impact on clinical care. Mt Sinai J Med 2009;76:111–8.

90. Liberzon I, Sripada CS. The functional neuroanatomy of PTSD: a critical review. Prog Brain Res 2008;167:151–69.

91. Rauch SL, Shin LM, Phelps EA. Neurocircuitry models of posttraumatic stress disorder and extinction: human neuroimaging research–past, present, and future. Biol Psychiatry 2006;60:376–82.

92. Koenigs M, Huey ED, Raymont V, et al. Focal brain damage protects against post-traumatic stress disorder in combat veterans. Nat Neurosci 2008;11:232–7.

93. McAllister TW. Psychopharmacological issues in the treatment of TBI and PTSD. Clin Neuropsychol 2009;23:1338–67.

94. Agoston DV, Gyorgy A, Eidelman O, et al. Proteomic biomarkers for blast neurotrauma: targeting cerebral edema, inflammation, and neuronal death cascades. J Neurotrauma 2009;26:901–11.

95. Svetlov SI, Larner SF, Kirk DR, et al. Biomarkers of blast-induced neurotrauma: profiling molecular and cellular mechanisms of blast brain injury. J Neurotrauma 2009;26:913–21.

96. Iverson GL, Langlois JA, McCrea MA, et al. Challenges associated with post-deployment screening for mild traumatic brain injury in military personnel. Clin Neuropsychol 2009;23:1299–314.

97. Jaffee MS, Meyer KS. A brief overview of traumatic brain injury (TBI) and post-traumatic stress disorder (PTSD) within the Department of Defense. Clin Neuropsychol 2009;23:1291–8.

98. Available at: www.dvbic.org. Accessed September 23, 2010.

99. Available at: http://www.defense.gov/news/newsarticle.aspx?id=58342. Accessed September 23, 2010.

100. Available at: http://www.polytrauma.va.gov/. Accessed September 23, 2010.
101. VA/DoD Clinical Practice Guideline for Management of Concussion/Mild Traumatic Brain Injury (mTBI) 2009. Available at: www.healthquality.va.gov/mtbi/concussion_mtbi_full_1_0.pdf. Accessed September 23, 2010.
102. Kaur C, Singh J, Lim MK, et al. Macrophages/microglia as 'sensors' of injury in the pineal gland of rats following a non-penetrative blast. Neurosci Res 1997;27:317–22.
103. Kaur C, Singh J, Lim MK, et al. The response of neurons and microglia to blast injury in the rat brain. Neuropathol Appl Neurobiol 1995;21:369–77.
104. Kaur C, Singh J, Lim MK, et al. Studies of the choroid plexus and its associated epiplexus cells in the lateral ventricles of rats following an exposure to a single non-penetrative blast. Arch Histol Cytol 1996;59:239–48.
105. Saljo A, Bao F, Haglid KG, et al. Blast exposure causes redistribution of phosphorylated neurofilament subunits in neurons of the adult rat brain. J Neurotrauma 2000;17:719–26.
106. Saljo A, Bao F, Hamberger A, et al. Exposure to short-lasting impulse noise causes microglial and astroglial cell activation in the adult rat brain. Pathophysiology 2001;8:105–11.
107. Saljo A, Bao F, Jingshan S, et al. Exposure to short-lasting impulse noise causes neuronal c-Jun expression and induction of apoptosis in the adult rat brain. J Neurotrauma 2002;19:985–91.
108. Saljo A, Bao F, Shi J, et al. Expression of c-Fos and c-Myc and deposition of beta-APP in neurons in the adult rat brain as a result of exposure to short-lasting impulse noise. J Neurotrauma 2002;19:379–85.
109. Kato K, Fujimura M, Nakagawa A, et al. Pressure-dependent effect of shock waves on rat brain: induction of neuronal apoptosis mediated by a caspase-dependent pathway. J Neurosurg 2007;106:667–76.

Combat-Related Traumatic Brain Injury and Its Implications to Military Healthcare

Kimberly S. Meyer, MSN, ACNP[a,b],*, Donald W. Marion, MD[a],
Helen Coronel, MSN, FNP[a], Michael S. Jaffee, MD[a]

KEYWORDS

• TBI • PTSD • Screening • Management

Casualties are common realities associated with combat. Fatalities from the Vietnam War are estimated to be 58,000.[1] Deaths resulting from Operation Enduring Freedom (OEF) and Operation Iraqi Freedom (OIF) are much lower, at 1070 and 4401, respectively,[2] and the current conflicts boast a significantly greater percentage of casualties surviving their injuries (OEF, 5917, and OIF, 31,822). The increase in survivability of combat-related injuries is attributed to improvements in body armor and advances in battlefield medicine. OEF and OIF have resulted in a large number of exposures to blast injury; the potential for blast waves resulting in traumatic brain injury (TBI) is an area of intense research (see the article by Elder and colleagues for further exploration of this topic). Confounding the diagnosis and management of patients with physical injuries is the psychological distress associated with operating in a combat theater. In a study of service members who sustained burns as a result of combat, 36% of the patients were diagnosed with posttraumatic stress disorder (PTSD) and 41% with mild TBI.[3] The challenge confronting military medicine is in diagnosing these conditions because neither mild TBI nor psychological disorders are readily recognized.

Recovery from TBI is related to several factors, including number of deployments and previous brain injuries and presence of co-occurring psychological distress, psychiatric comorbidities, pain syndromes, and other medical illnesses. Recently, increased awareness of both TBI and its neurobehavioral sequelae has resulted in a change in the military's policies related to casualty management. This article

[a] Defense and Veterans Brain Injury Center, PO Box 59181, Washington, DC 20012, USA
[b] University of Louisville Hospital, Trauma Institute, 530 South Jackson Street, Louisville, KY 40202, USA
* Corresponding author.
E-mail address: kimberly.meyer1@us.army.mil

Psychiatr Clin N Am 33 (2010) 783–796
doi:10.1016/j.psc.2010.08.007
0193-953X/10/$ – see front matter © 2010 Elsevier Inc. All rights reserved.

summarizes these changes and the current efforts related to identifying and caring for soldiers with TBI.

DEFINITION OF TBI

The Department of Defense (DoD) policy defines TBI as a traumatically induced structural injury and/or physiologic disruption of brain function as a result of an external force that is indicated by one or more new or worsening clinical signs immediately after the event.[4] These clinical signs include

- Any period of loss or decreased level of consciousness
- Loss of memory for events before or after the injury
- Alteration in mental state at the time of injury
- Neurologic deficits or intracranial lesion.

This definition is consistent with other definitions presented by the Centers for Disease Control, World Health Organization, and American Congress of Rehabilitation Medicine. TBI is actually a spectrum of injuries ranging from mild TBI, in which outcomes are generally excellent, to severe TBI, in which the mortality can approach 30%. Appropriate classification of the severity of injury is important because it is prognostic of functional recovery, resource allocation, and expected long-term sequelae.

PATHOPHYSIOLOGY OF COMBAT-RELATED TBI

In civilian settings, TBI is most often caused by blunt traumatic forces. In today's combat setting, TBI is often attributed to blast injury or a combination of blast and blunt trauma. Exposure to blast may result in brain injury through several mechanisms:

- Primary injuries resulting from rapid changes in air pressure after the explosion
- Secondary injuries resulting from debris that has been set in motion by explosive forces
- Tertiary injuries resulting from kinetic forces of an individual being set in motion by blast forces and subsequent deceleration
- Quaternary injuries sustained as a result of heat or noxious fumes.

Much of the data regarding evaluation and treatment modalities for TBI are based on blunt trauma, particularly sports-related injury. However, emerging evidence demonstrates that there may be pathophysiologic differences between blunt and blast brain injuries as evidenced by abnormalities in fractional anisotropy on diffusion tensor imaging,[5] even in mild TBI. Armonda and colleagues[6] have shown that people affected by severe TBI caused by blasts have a higher incidence of developing vasospasm and pseudoaneurysm than that previously identified in civilian populations. Despite these pathologic differences, there is no convincing evidence that the sequelae or disability vary by cause of injury.[7]

TBI SCREENING IN DOD

Since 2000, a total of 169,838 service members have sustained a TBI.[8] More than 80% of these injuries are categorized as concussion or mild TBI, reflective of only a brief alteration or loss of consciousness (LOC). Aggressive screening measures were instituted in 2006 to ensure that this population with mild TBI, who generally return to normal functional levels within hours to days, is captured in military TBI surveillance. Screening occurs in a variety of settings across the continuum of care, beginning in the combat theater. After exposure to a traumatic event, injured service members undergo evaluation using the Military Acute Concussion Evaluation (MACE) (**Fig. 1**). The MACE has 3 domains: description of the traumatic event, symptoms, and cognitive function using the Standardized Assessment of Concussion.[9] More recently, efforts to screen all service members exposed to blast injury immediately after the event, regardless of the appearance of symptoms, have been initiated. Additional screening occurs for all service members medically evacuated from the combat

Military Acute Concussion Evaluation (MACE)

Patient Name: _____

SS#: _____-_____-_____ Unit: _____

Date of Injury: ____/____/____ Time of Injury: _____

Examiner: _____

Date of Evaluation: ____/____/____ Time of Evaluation: _____

History: (I – IX)

I. **Description of Incident**
Ask:
A) What happened?
B) Tell me what you remember.
C) Were you dazed, confused, "saw stars"? ❑ Yes ❑ No
D) Did you hit your head? ❑ Yes ❑ No

II. **Cause of Injury** (Circle all that apply):
1) Explosion/Blast   4) Fragment
2) Blunt Object   5) Fall
3) Motor Vehicle Crash   6) Gunshot wound
7) Other _____

III. **Was a helmet worn?** ❑ Yes ❑ No   Type _____

IV. **Amnesia Before: Are there any events just BEFORE the injury that are not remembered?**
(Assess for continuous memory prior to injury.)
❑ Yes ❑ No If yes, how long _____

V. **Amnesia After: Are there any events just AFTER the injuries that are not remembered?**
(Assess time until continuous memory after the injury.)
❑ Yes ❑ No If yes, how long _____

VI. **Does the individual report loss of consciousness or "blacking out"?** ❑ Yes ❑ No If yes, how long _____

VII. **Did anyone observe a period of loss of consciousness or unresponsiveness?** ❑ Yes ❑ No If yes, how long _____

VIII. **Have you had any concussions in the last 12 months?**
❑ Yes ❑ No If yes, how long _____

IX. **Symptoms** (circle all that apply)
1) Headache   6) Difficulty Concentrating
2) Dizziness   7) Irritability
3) Memory Problems   8) Visual Disturbances
4) Balance Problems   9) Ringing in the Ears
5) Nausea/Vomiting   10) Other_____

Symptom Score:
A(no current symptoms) / B(one or more current symptoms)

01/2010   DVBIC.org   800-870-9244
This form may be copied for clinical use.
Page 1 of 8

Fig. 1. Military Acute Concussion Evaluation. (*Courtesy of* the Defense and Veterans Brain Injury Center, Washington, DC.)

theater through Landstuhl Regional Medical Center (LRMC).[10] Using this process, 20% to 25% of patients screen positive for TBI. Also, service members can self-report exposure to a traumatic event with subsequent alteration or LOC and any ongoing symptoms in the Postdeployment Health Assessment, a mandatory health question-naire required on return from a combat rotation. Positive screens are then referred to a provider for an in-depth interview and examination before a formal diagnosis of TBI is made. One study demonstrated that 22.8% of soldiers returning from Iraq had sustained a clinician-confirmed TBI during their deployment. In this population, 33.4% of soldiers reported 3 or more symptoms immediately after the injury and this decreased to 7.5% by postdeployment.[11]

MANAGEMENT OF COMBAT-RELATED TBI

Identification of severe and penetrating TBI occurs rapidly based on physical exami-nation and prompts rapid triage and transport to designated trauma-support facilities. Although comprising only a small percentage of combat-related TBI, this population is resource-intensive, with the potential for acute changes in the neurologic condition. Unpublished data from the Defense and Veterans Brain Injury Center (2009) suggest that the severity of TBI in the military is similar to that in civilian populations, 4% severe, 4% penetrating, and 8% moderate. As a result, patients with this type of injury are rapidly stabilized and evacuated stateside to Walter Reed Army Medical Center or National Naval Medical Center, after only a brief stop at LRMC for further resuscitation and stabilization. Overall, management is in accordance with the Guidelines for the Surgical Management of Traumatic Brain Injury[12] and the Guidelines for the Manage-ment of Severe Traumatic Brain Injury, third edition.[13]

As previously stated, most combat-related TBIs are categorized as mild or concus-sive injuries. There are few well-designed studies to guide the care of these patients, especially in the acute setting. Management occurs in a primary care setting, with education and expectation of recovery at the forefront of the treatment plan. Provision of such materials is one of the few interventions shown to decrease symptom report-ing in patients with mild TBI (**Box 1**).[14] Postconcussive symptoms are monitored using Cicerone's Neurobehavioral Symptom Inventory (**Fig. 2**).[15,16] This inventory provides a tool to monitor symptom progression and resolution, whereas consensus-based clinical practice guidelines provide a framework to evaluate and manage symptoms, given the resource limitations that can exist in combat settings. Predominant physical complaints reported in multiple military samples include headache, dizziness, and balance problems, along with other less common somatosensory disruptions.[11] Cognitive and behavioral complaints are also prevalent and include memory and attention deficits, sleep disturbances, and mood symptoms.[17] Unpublished DoD data suggest that service members evaluated and treated using these guidelines immediately after a single concussion have symptom resolution, allowing them to return to duty (RTD) within 3 weeks of injury.

In addition to providing education regarding the natural history of concussion recovery, injured service members are placed on restricted duty to facilitate rest and recovery. Headache, the predominant symptom, is managed using immediate treatment with acetaminophen. If the headache persists for more than a week, prophylactic medications such as amitriptyline are initiated. Once symptoms are controlled, exertional testing is performed to determine if symptoms or cognitive dysfunction recur with physical activity. In-theater management continues for 2 weeks after the injury; patients with resolving symptoms may be monitored slightly longer. Evacuation is considered for those injured service members who fail to respond to initial management. Current DoD policy requires a comprehensive evaluation for all service members sustaining 3 or more concussions within a 12-month period. This comprehensive evaluation includes detailed neurologic and psychological evaluations, as well as balance and visual screening.

Once stateside, patients with persistent symptoms or those who did not receive short-term TBI care are managed using the Veterans Affairs (VA)/DoD Evidence Based Guideline: Management of Concussion/Mild Traumatic Brain Injury[18] published in 2009. In addition to symptom management, these algorithms focus on sleep hygiene, relaxation, and self-management techniques that are often impractical to use in a combat setting. As a result of combat-related injuries, vague complaints of visual dysfunction and dizziness, which traditionally have been dismissed, have been scientifically evaluated. In a retrospective study of 192 combat-injured service members with TBI of all severities, Brahm and colleagues[19] found that a significant number of patients treated at a VA polytrauma rehabilitation center had accommodation insufficiency (40%) or convergence insufficiency (43%). Loss of visual acuity and field cuts were seen predominantly in those with moderate to severe injury. These findings were not statistically significant for blast versus blunt trauma and, therefore, may affect civilian TBI care. In contrast, blast injury may cause unique vestibular dysfunction, which may continue into the long-term recovery.[20] Dynamic balance testing and auditory testing objectively identify deficits in vestibular function, which have been shown to worsen with time.

MILD TBI AND COEXISTING CONDITIONS

There is a complex and unclear interface between postconcussive symptoms attributed to brain injury and PTSD or other behavioral sequelae of having been in a psychologically stressful situation or secondary to an underlying predisposing vulnerability to these conditions. It is generally accepted that there are somatic symptoms associated with mild TBI, but there is accumulating evidence that persistent symptoms after reasonable treatment may be attributable to emotional distress or to possible preexisting psychiatric comorbidities.[21,22] Boake and colleagues[23] have reported that there is a small subset of patients with mild and moderate TBI in the civilian setting, who are unable to return to work at 6 months after injury. The investigators compared 210 patients with mild to moderate TBI and 122 general trauma patients without TBI. Reasons cited for difficulties with employment did not include specific symptoms, although vague reasons were reported, such as feeling under pressure and having difficulty remembering or concentrating. Postconcussive symptoms are diagnosed immediately in up to 43% of those with mild TBI, although at least one study found that postconcussive type symptoms are also common in trauma patients without TBI.[24] More than 80% of these injuries are categorized as concussion or mild TBI, reflective of only a brief alteration or LOC.

The diagnosis of postconcussive syndrome (PCS) is often inappropriately made based on isolated symptoms occurring in the acute phase of injury. The World Health Organization requires the presence of 3 or more of the following 8 symptoms for classification of PCS: (1) headache, (2) dizziness, (3) fatigue, (4) irritability, (5) insomnia, (6) concentration, (7) memory difficulty, and (8) intolerance of stress, emotion, or alcohol.[25] Both the *International Classification of Diseases Tenth Revision* and the *Diagnostic Statistical Manual of Mental Disorders* (Fourth Edition) require a temporal relationship of symptom onset with traumatic event and prolonged duration of symptoms before diagnosing PCS. PCS is common among service members who

---

Box 1
Concussion/mild TBI information: at the time of injury (acute)

What happened to me? Your assessment indicates that you have had a concussion, which is also called a "mild traumatic brain injury"

What is a concussion? A concussion is a head injury from a hit, blow, or jolt to the head that briefly knocks you out (LOC) or makes you feel confused or "see stars" (alteration or change in consciousness)

- Immediately or soon after the concussion, you may have disorientation, headaches, dizziness, balance difficulties, ringing in the ears, blurred vision, nausea, vomiting, irritability, temporary gaps in your memory, sleep problems, or attention and concentration problems

How Long Does It Last? Most people recover from concussion

- Symptoms usually begin to improve within hours and typically resolve completely within days to weeks
- Even if you've had more than 1 concussion, full recovery is expected. However, every time you sustain an additional concussion, your healing might take longer

Recovery

- Recovery is different for each person and depends on the nature of the injury
- The most important thing you can do is to allow time for your brain to heal
- Be honest about your symptoms and let your medical provider decide when it is time to RTD

Why does a concussion affect RTD?

- Often after a concussion, service members think that they are alright, yet they have actually had an injury that needs attention
- Symptoms after concussion reduce your effectiveness, which could impair your performance and endanger your mission

    These temporary impairments resolve fastest when your brain gets rest (similar to resting a sprained ankle)

- If you get another concussion before healing from the first one, you are at a greater risk for a more serious injury

Healing from a concussion

Things that improve healing

- Maximize downtime/rest during the day
- Get plenty of sleep at night
- Protect yourself from another concussion: avoid contact sports, combatives, and other similar physical activities
- Let others know that you have had a concussion so that they can watch out for you
- Return immediately to your medical provider if you are feeling worse or experiencing any of the warning signs*

Things that impair healing

- Another concussion before healing from the first one
- Alcohol and drug use
- Inadequate sleep (made worse by caffeine or energy-enhancing products)
- Aspirin, ibuprofen, and other over-the-counter pain medications unless instructed by your doctor
- Sleeping aids and sedatives unless instructed by your doctor

What are your medical instructions now that you have been diagnosed with a concussion?

- You have already reported it and been checked out

  Be honest with your providers (they are protecting you and your unit)

- Rest

  Avoid exerting yourself physically (eg, working, heavy lifting, exercising)

  Avoid mental exertion (eg, writing reports, thinking, activities requiring you to pay attention)

- RTD

  Expect to recover fully and RTD

  Your provider will continue to evaluate you and will determine when it is safe for you to RTD

Additional information: Defense and Veterans Brain injury Center. http://www.dvbic.org. Developed by Battlemind Transition Office and Proponency Office for Rehabilitation and Reintegration, Version 4.0, 27 May, 2010.
* Warning Signs: If you begin to experience any of the following, seek immediate medical attention: worsening headache, worsening balance, double vision or other vision changes, decreasing level of alertness, increased disorientation, repeated vomiting, seizures, unusual behavior, amnesia/memory problems.

experience TBI, although there is no clear evidence that it is more common among those exposed to blast injury compared with those with TBI from other mechanisms.[26] In civilian studies, motor vehicle crash or assault as the mechanism of injury, female gender, and a premorbid history of affective or anxiety disorders are risk factors for development of PCS.[24,27,28]

The presence of one or more of these postconcussive symptoms may affect job performance in the combat arena. Marksmanship can be impaired by visual disturbances, dizziness, and balance problems. Fatigue, concentration difficulties, and memory problems have the potential to diminish situational awareness and the ability to carry out mission orders. For these reasons, everyone involved in traumatic events of specified magnitude undergo TBI screening. In some circumstances, functional assessments or closely supervised duties are necessary to ensure the safety and welfare of the team.

In a study of 2525 soldiers returning from ground combat in Iraq, 4.9% sustained TBI with LOC and 10.3%, TBI with alteration of consciousness (AOC).[17] Of the patients with LOC and AOC, 43.9% and 27.3%, respectively, met criteria for PTSD. Missed work days and increased symptom reporting occurred significantly more often in those with mild TBI compared with those in the sample who sustained injuries other than brain injury and those without any documented injury. Physical symptoms were reported using the patient health questionnaire -15. Of note, only headache was found to be specific to mild TBI. The incidence of mild TBI described by Hoge and colleagues[17] is similar to that reported by Wilk and colleagues.[29]

Chronic pain is also a common comorbidity associated with TBI. To better understand the risk factors and characteristics of pain associated with TBI, Nampiaparampil[30] reviewed all relevant studies from 1951 to 2008. According to 12 studies that described 1670 patients with TBI, the prevalence of headache was approximately 57.8% at 3 months or longer after injury. The prevalence of chronic pain of unspecified

Neurobehavioral Symptom Inventory					
Please rate the following symptoms with regard to how much they have disturbed you IN THE LAST 2 Weeks.					
0 = None – Rarely if ever present; not a problem at all					
1 = Mild – Occasionally present, but it does not disrupt my activities; I can usually continue what I'm doing; doesn't really concern me.					
2 = Moderate – Often present, occasionally disrupts my activities; I can usually continue what I'm doing with some effort; I feel somewhat concerned.					
3 = Severe – Frequently present and disrupts activities; I can only do things that are fairly simple or take little effort; I feel I need help.					
4 = Very Severe – Almost always present and I have been unable to perform at work, school or home due to this problem, I probably cannot function without help.					

Symptoms	0	1	2	3	4
Feeling Dizzy	O	O	O	O	O
Loss of balance	O	O	O	O	O
Poor coordination, clumsy	O	O	O	O	O
Headaches	O	O	O	O	O
Nausea	O	O	O	O	O
Vision problems, blurring, trouble seeing	O	O	O	O	O
Sensitivity to light	O	O	O	O	O
Hearing difficulty	O	O	O	O	O
Sensitivity to noise	O	O	O	O	O
Numbness or tingling on parts of my body	O	O	O	O	O
Change in taste and/or smell	O	O	O	O	O
Loss of appetite or increased appetite	O	O	O	O	O
Poor concentration, can't pay attention, easily distracted	O	O	O	O	O
Forgetfulness, can't remember things	O	O	O	O	O
Difficulty making decisions	O	O	O	O	O
Slowed thinking, difficulty getting organized, can't finish things	O	O	O	O	O
Fatigue, loss of energy, getting tired easily	O	O	O	O	O
Difficulty falling or staying asleep	O	O	O	O	O
Feeling anxious or tense	O	O	O	O	O
Feeling depressed or sad	O	O	O	O	O
Irritability, easily annoyed	O	O	O	O	O
Poor frustration tolerance, feeling easily overwhelmed by things	O	O	O	O	O

PT Name _____ Clinician_____

ID _____ Date _____

Fig. 2. Neurobehavioral symptom inventory. (*From* Cicerone KD, Kalmar K. Persistent post-concussion syndrome: the structure of subjective complaints after mild traumatic brain injury. J Head Trauma Rehabil 1995;10:1–17; with permission.)

cause was 51.5% based on 20 studies describing 3289 patients with TBI. Chronic pain was much more prevalent with mild TBI (75.3%) than with moderate or severe TBI (32.1%). In 917 veterans with a history of TBI, the prevalence of chronic pain was 43.1%. This study also found that chronic pain occurred independently of PTSD or depression, a conclusion that somewhat conflicts with the findings of others.[31] Higher incidences of chronic pain were found (81.5%) in a cohort of 340 OIF or OEF veterans who screened positive for mild TBI at a VA Polytrauma Network Site, with most of the pain reported in the head and back. In this study, although pain did occur independently, chronic pain, persistent postconcussive symptoms, and PTSD coexisted in most cases (42.1%).[32]

Headache is one of the most prominent symptoms of TBI, found to be as high as 97% by Theeler and colleagues.[32] Posttraumatic headaches were found to contribute to more loss-of-duty time than other types of headache. Acute posttraumatic headaches begin within 2 weeks of injury and usually resolve in a similar time frame. Headaches persisting longer than 8 weeks are considered to be chronic. These chronic headaches are typically described as migrainous or tension-type.[33,34]

Excessive sleepiness is also commonly reported by patients after a mild TBI. In a study of 689 patients with mild TBI compared with 1318 patients without TBI, Kraus and colleagues[35] used the Pittsburgh Sleep Quality Index to assess sleep quality overall, sleep latency, and daytime sleepiness and reported a significant decrement in the mild TBI group. In a study by Castriotta and colleagues,[36] 46% of the patients with mild TBI had sleep abnormalities 3 months after injury; 25% had objective evidence of excessive daytime sleepiness. Although TBI is associated with a variety of sleep disorders, including insomnia and parasomnia, the most common disorder is hypersomnia.[37] Whether excessive sleepiness is specific to TBI or is a result of trauma in general is controversial. One prospective study of 524 subjects with TBI and 132 noncranial trauma patients found excessive sleepiness (1 or more sleepiness items on the Sickness Impact Profile) not only in 55% of subjects with TBI but also in 41% noncranial trauma patients.[38] Subjective fatigue is also common after TBI but seems unrelated to injury severity, time after injury, degree of cognitive impairment, or gender.[39] Although these studies reflect the findings in civilian populations, similar sleep disturbances have been noted in symptom inventories in military populations.[17]

A variety of psychiatric disorders are more common in those who have experienced a TBI than in those who have not.[40] Silver and colleagues[41] studied 5034 adults from New Haven, Connecticut, and found that 361 admitted to a history of TBI with LOC or confusion. Compared to subjects without TBI, those with TBI were at an increased risk for major depression, dysthymia, panic disorder, obsessive-compulsive disorder, phobic disorder, drug abuse and dependence, and lifetime risk of suicide attempts when controlled for socioeconomic factors, quality-of-life indicators, and alcohol use. Depression is a common condition associated with TBI, and this association is of heightened concern in the military because of the recent reports of an increase in the number of suicides. Jorge and colleagues[42] investigated the association between major depression and TBI in a prospective study of 91 patients with TBI compared with 27 control subjects with non–central nervous system (CNS) trauma. The investigators found that 52% of the subjects with TBI developed a mood disorder within 1 year of injury, 33% of whom had major depressive disorders, and that this rate was significantly higher than that for the control subjects. Patients with TBI and depression were more likely to have a pre-TBI history of mood and anxiety disorders. After TBI, patients with major depression also were more likely to have anxiety, aggressive behavior, impaired executive functions, and poorer social functioning. Those who were depressed had a lower score in neuropsychological testing related to attention and executive function as well as decreased left frontal gray matter volumes at the 3-month evaluation.

There are several case reports, mostly in public media sources, of suicides by OIF and OEF veterans. Although there is often an implied link between suicide and TBI in active-duty service members and veterans, no true correlation has been established. In a small study of veterans with a history of TBI and suicide attempts, participants identified loss of sense of self, cognitive difficulties, and emotional distress after their injury as contributing factors to their suicide attempt.[43]

Substance abuse is a well-recognized risk factor for TBI, but most studies find that substance abuse rates actually decline after a TBI, including mild TBI.[44] Preinjury alcohol and drug misuse are the most important predictors for postinjury abuse.

Veterans with a history of problematic drug or alcohol use before injury were more likely to require inpatient psychiatric treatment within the first 10 years after TBI compared with a similar group with TBI and without known substance misuse history.[45] In addition, substance abuse is more common among subjects with mild TBI who are unemployed and among those with mood disorders.[46] This same study found impaired executive functioning and decreased volume of medial frontal gray matter volumes, a finding worthy of further investigation because this may contribute to vocational difficulties.

PTSD is increasingly recognized as a complication of a variety of traumatic events, including TBI.[47] Most investigators agree that the development of this disorder must involve some memory of the traumatic event and that PTSD is manifested as some combination of 3 symptom clusters: reexperience, avoidance, or hyperarousal. The importance of the memory of the event is emphasized by a study of 120 patients with mild TBI, which found that those who regained memory of the traumatic event within the first 24 hours after the trauma were significantly more likely to develop PTSD than those with posttraumatic amnesia for 24 hours or more.[48] Indeed, PTSD is unlikely to occur if TBI is associated with an extended period of LOC. In a study of 46 patients referred to a neurologic rehabilitation clinic for sequelae of TBI, Glaesser and colleagues,[49] found PTSD in 3% (1 of 31 patients) of those unconscious for more than 12 hours but in 27% of those not unconscious "for an extended period." The most common symptom clusters were intrusive memories and reexperiencing symptoms. Some studies have also defined specific mechanisms of injury and other characteristics that seem to increase the risk for the development of PTSD after TBI. Hill and colleagues[50] evaluated 94 service members who had positive TBI screens and were deployed between April 2007 and March 2008 and found that 85% of the subjects had probable mild TBI as defined by the American Congress of Rehabilitation Medicine. Compared with service members who had only TBI, those with PTSD and TBI were more likely to report falling as a mechanism and relate that they had experienced TBI during deployment and had more exposures and symptoms. In a cross-sectional cohort study of Vietnam War veterans, mild TBI was found to be associated with headaches, memory problems, sleep problems, and fainting despite controlling for psychiatric conditions such as PTSD. The study also found that mild TBI adversely affected the long-term outcomes of PTSD treatment.[51] The poor understanding of TBI during the Vietnam War era may explain the difficulties with adequate treatment of PTSD in this population. Further research is needed to determine if aggressive management of TBI and its associated symptoms affects the overall outcome of PTSD treatment.

NEUROPSYCHOLOGICAL TESTING

Given the need to preserve the fighting force while ensuring the safety of individual service members, careful consideration for RTD after TBI is warranted. Part of this evaluation may include a brief neuropsychological screen using the Automated Neuropsychological Assessment Metrics (ANAM). This computerized battery test includes measures of reaction times, memory, and mathematical processing. After injury, the ANAM is administered, and results are compared with the individual's baseline to screen for new cognitive deficits that may delay return to full duty. Efforts to expand the use of the ANAM to routine postdeployment screening stalled when a study of 956 soldiers returning from OIF/OEF demonstrated that a history of self-reported TBI during the deployment did not result in cognitive deficits.[52] This finding may be the result of a brief neuropsychological screening battery that is not adequately sensitive. Scientific evaluation of other neuropsychological screening tests in a head-to-head study is underway. Findings from this study will help determine the optimal postinjury screening tool.

RESEARCH OPPORTUNITIES

Highlighting the importance of TBI, $40.6 million were allocated for psychological health and TBI research initiatives for the fiscal year 2010 disbursement through the Congressionally Directed Medical Research Programs (CDMRP). Some areas of funding interest are

- Military-related psychological health issues
- Cellular regrowth and interconnection strategies and therapies for the CNS
- Evidence-based prevention and rehabilitation strategies for TBI, PTSD, and other co-occurring conditions
- Three-dimensional models of blast waves of improvised explosive devices to develop injury mitigation strategies
- Advanced neuroimaging, biomarkers, behavioral or genetic information, and advanced computational research to better understand the intersection of psychological health and TBI.

Funded projects will further augment work being performed at the Center for Neuroscience and Regenerative Medicine at the Uniformed Services University of the Health Sciences, the Armed Forces Institute of Pathology, and other DoD research facilities. Other studies currently in progress include

- Neuroendocrine studies: Studies are evaluating the hypothalamic-pituitary-adrenal (HPA) axis in blast-related TBI and PTSD to determine the incidence and variability in HPA dysfunction. Previous data from blunt injury demonstrate differences in hormonal function between patients with TBI and PTSD
- Longitudinal study of mild TBI: This study is to evaluate the validity of the screening tool used by the DoD and VA and to better understand the long-term interactions between TBI and psychological symptoms
- CDMRP studies are being conducted on the effects of blast waves on biologic and CNS tissue
- Helmet-mounted sensor study: A sensor prototype is being evaluated by the Army Medical Research and Materiel Command. These sensors detect blast exposure and aid in TBI risk assessment in service members in high-risk occupations
- Institute of Soldier Nanotechnology (ISN): DVBIC is collaborating on several projects with ISN at the Massachusetts Institute of Technology to include the development of the most advanced system of computer modeling of blast effects on the brain.

SUMMARY

Management of combat-related TBI is complicated by several factors including the resource limitations in a combat setting, poorly understood effects of blast brain injury, effects of cumulative concussion, and presence of co-occurring psychological, psychiatric, and medical comorbidities. Current efforts aimed at understanding the interaction between TBI and psychological/psychiatric conditions should continue. Further research is needed to determine the pathophysiologic basis of the symptoms of TBI and comorbid psychological disorders. In the interim, symptom management should prevail.

REFERENCES

1. Available at: http://www.archives.gov/research/vietnam-war/casualty-statistics. html. Accessed April 28, 2010.
2. Available at: http://www.defense.gov/news/casualty.pdf. Accessed April 28, 2010.
3. Gaylord KM, Cooper DB, Mercado JB, et al. Incidence of post-traumatic stress disorder and mild traumatic brain injury in burned service members: a preliminary report. J Trauma 2008;64(Suppl 2):S200–5.
4. HA Policy 07-030. Traumatic brain injury: definition and reporting. Memorandum from the Assistant Secretary of Defense for Health Affairs. October 1, 2007.
5. Warden DL, French LM, Shupenko I , et al. Case report of a soldier with primary blast brain injury. Neuroimage 2009;47(Suppl 2):T152–3.
6. Armonda RA, Bell RS, Vo AH, et al. Wartime traumatic cerebral vasospasm: recent review of combat casualties. Neurosurgery 2006;59:1215–25.
7. Belanger H, Kretzmer T, Yoash-Gantz R, et al. Cognitive sequelae of blast-related brain trauma versus other mechanisms of brain trauma. J Int Neuropsychol Soc 2009;15:1–8.
8. Available at: http://www.dvbic.org/TBI-Numbers.aspx. Accessed April 28, 2010.
9. McCrea M, Kelly J, Randolph C. Standardized Assessment of Concussion (SAC): manual for administration, scoring, and interpretation. 2nd edition. Waukesha (WI): Comprehensive Neuropsychological Services; 2000.
10. Dempsey KE, Dorlac WC, Martin K, et al. Landstuhl Regional Medical Center: traumatic brain injury screening program. J Trauma Nurs 2009;16:6–12.
11. Terrio H, Brenner LA, Ivins BJ, et al. Traumatic brain injury screening: preliminary findings in a US army brigade combat team. J Head Trauma Rehabil 2009;24: 14–23.
12. Brain Trauma Foundation. American Association of Neurological Surgeons; Congress of Neurological Surgeons; Joint Section on Neurotrauma and Critical Care, AANS/CNS. Guidelines for the management of severe traumatic brain injury. J Neurotrauma 2007;24(Suppl 1):1–90.
13. Brain Trauma Foundation. American Association of Neurological Surgeons; Congress of Neurological Surgeons. Guidelines for the management of penetrating brain injury. J Trauma 2001;51(Suppl 2):S3.
14. Ponsford J. Rehabilitation interventions after mild head injury. Curr Opin Neurol 2005;18:692–7.
15. Kennedy JE, Cullen MA, Amador RR, et al. Symptoms in military service members after blast mTBI with and without associated injuries. NeuroRehabilitation 2010;26:191–7.
16. Cicerone KD, Kalmar K. Persistent post-concussion syndrome: the structure of subjective complaints after mild traumatic brain injury. J Head Trauma Rehabil 1995;10:1–17.
17. Hoge CW, McGurk D, Thomas JL, et al. Mild traumatic brain injury in US soldiers returning from Iraq. N Engl J Med 2008;358:453–63.
18. Available at: http://www.healthquality.va.gov/mtbi/concussion_mtbi_full_1_0.pdf. Accessed May 27, 2010.
19. Brahm KD, Wilgenburg HM, Kirby J, et al. Visual impairment and dysfunction in combat-injured service members with traumatic brain injury. Optom Vis Sci 2009;86:817–25.
20. Hoffer ME, Balaban C, Gottshall K, et al. Blast-exposure: vestibular consequences and associated characteristics. Otol Neurotol 2010;31:232–6.

21. Belanger HG, Kretzmer T, Vanderploeg RD, et al. Symptom complaints following combat-related traumatic brain injury: relationship to traumatic brain injury severity and posttraumatic stress disorder. J Int Neuropsychol Soc 2010;16:194–9.
22. Benge JF, Pastorek NJ, Thornton GM. Postconcussive symptoms in OEF-OIF veterans: factor structure and impact of posttraumatic stress. Rehabil Psychol 2009;54:270.
23. Boake C, McCauley SR, Pedroza C, et al. Lost productive work time after mild to moderate traumatic brain injury with and without hospitalization. Neurosurgery 2005;56:994–1003.
24. Meares S, Shores EA, Taylor AJ, et al. Mild traumatic brain injury does not predict acute postconcussion syndrome. J Neurol Neurosurg Psychiatr 2008; 79:300–6.
25. Halbauer J, Ashford J, Zeitzer J, et al. Neuropsychiatric diagnosis and management of chronic sequelae of war-related mild to moderate traumatic brain injury. J Rehabil Res Dev 2009;46:757–95.
26. Fear NT, Jones E, Groom M, et al. Symptoms of post-concussional syndrome are non-specifically related to mild traumatic brain injury in UK Armed Forces personnel on return from deployment in Iraq: an analysis of self-reported data. Psychol Med 2009;39:1379–87.
27. Jakola AS, Müller K, Larsen M, et al. Five-year outcome after mild head injury: a prospective controlled study. Acta Neurol Scand 2007;115:398–402.
28. McCauley SR, Boake C, Levin HS, et al. Postconcussional disorder following mild to moderate traumatic brain injury: anxiety, depression, and social support as risk factors and comorbidities. J Clin Exp Neuropsychol 2001;23:792–808.
29. Wilk JE, Thomas JL, McGurk DM, et al. Mild traumatic brain injury (concussion) during combat: lack of association of blast mechanism with persistent postconcussive symptoms. J Head Trauma Rehabil 2010;25:9–14.
30. Nampiaparampil DE. Prevalence of chronic pain after traumatic brain injury: a systematic review. JAMA 2008;300:711–9.
31. Dobscha SK, Clark ME, Morasco BJ, et al. Systematic review of the literature on pain in patients with polytrauma including traumatic brain injury. Pain Med 2009; 10:1200–17.
32. Theeler BJ, Flynn FG, Erickson J. Headaches after concussion in US soldiers returning from Iraq or Afghanistan. Headache 2010. [Epub ahead of print].
33. Lew HL, Otis JD, Tun C, et al. Prevalence of chronic pain, posttraumatic stress disorder, and persistent postconcussive symptoms in OIF/OEF veterans: polytrauma clinical triad. J Rehabil Res Dev 2009;46:697–702.
34. Lew HL, Pei-Hsin L, Jong-Ling F, et al. Characteristics and treatment of headache after traumatic brain injury: a focused review. J Rehabil Res Dev 2006;85:619–27.
35. Kraus J, Hsu P, Schaffer K, et al. Pre-injury factors and 3-month outcomes following emergency department diagnosis of mild traumatic brain injury. J Head Trauma Rehabil 2009;24:344–54.
36. Castriotta RJ, Atanasov S, Wilde MC, et al. Treatment of sleep disorders after traumatic brain injury. J Clin Sleep Med 2009;5:137–44.
37. Verma A, Anand V, Verma NP. Sleep disorders in chronic traumatic brain injury. J Clin Sleep Med 2007;3:357–62.
38. Watson NF, Dikmen S, Machamer J, et al. Hypersomnia following traumatic brain Injury. J Clin Sleep Med 2007;3:363–8.
39. Borgaro SR, Baker J, Wethe JV, et al. Subjective reports of fatigue during early recovery from traumatic brain injury. J Head Trauma Rehabil 2005;20: 416–25.

40. Rogers JM, Read CA. Psychiatric comorbidities following traumatic brain injury. Brain Inj 2007;21:1321–33.
41. Silver JM, Kramer R, Greenwald S, et al. The association between head injuries and psychiatric disorders: findings from the New Haven NIMH Epidemiologic Catchment Area study. Brain Inj 2001;15:935–45.
42. Jorge RE, Robinson RG, Moser D, et al. Major depression following traumatic brain injury. Arch Gen Psychiatry 2001;61:42–50.
43. Brenner LA, Homaifar BY, Adler LE, et al. Suicidality and veterans with a history of traumatic brain injury. Rehabil Psychol 2009;54:390–7.
44. Graham DP, Cardon AL. An update on substance use and treatment following traumatic brain injury. Ann N Y Acad Sci 2008;1141:148–62.
45. Brenner LA, Harwood JE, Homaifar BY, et al. Psychiatric hospitalization and veterans with traumatic brain injury: a retrospective study. J Head Trauma Rehabil 2008;23:401–6.
46. Jorge JE, Starkstein SE, Arndt S, et al. Alcohol misuse and mood disorders following traumatic brain injury. Arch Gen Psychiatry 2005;62:742–9.
47. Pietrzak RH, Johnson DC, Goldstein MB, et al. Posttraumatic stress disorder mediates the relationship between mild traumatic brain injury and health and psychosocial functioning in veterans of Operations Enduring Freedom and Iraqi Freedom. J Nerv Ment Dis 2009;197:748–53.
48. Gil S, Caspi S, Ben-Ari IZ, et al. Does memory of a traumatic event increase the risk of post-traumatic stress disorder in patients with traumatic brain injury. Am J Psychiatry 2005;162:963–9.
49. Glaesser J, Neuner F, Lutgehetmann R, et al. Post-traumatic stress disorder in patients with traumatic brain injury. BMC Psychiatry 2004;9:5.
50. Hill JJ 3rd, Mobo BH Jr, Cullen MR. Separating deployment-related traumatic brain injury and post-traumatic stress disorder in veterans: preliminary findings from the Veterans Affairs traumatic brain injury screening program. Am J Phys Med Rehabil 2009;88:605–14.
51. Vanderploeg RD, Belanger HG, Curtiss G. Mild traumatic brain injury and post-traumatic stress disorder and their associations with health symptoms. Arch Phys Med Rehabil 2009;90:1084–93.
52. Ivins BJ, Kane R, Schwab KA. Performance on the automated neuropsychological assessment metrics in a nonclinical sample of soldiers screened for mild traumatic brain injury after returning from Iraq and Afghanistan: a descriptive analysis. J Head Trauma Rehabil 2009;24:24–31.

Mild Traumatic Brain Injury: Key Decisions in Acute Management

Andy S. Jagoda, MD

KEYWORDS

• Mild traumatic brain injury • Postconcussive disorders
• Rehabilitation • Neurobehavioral • Sequelae

Mild traumatic brain injury (TMI) has historically been defined as an injury to the head, with or without loss of consciousness, and a Glasgow Coma Scale Score (GCS) of 13 to 15. It is estimated that in the United States there are between 1 and 2 million patients evaluated in emergency departments (EDs) for a mild TBI.[1] Falls and motor vehicle crashes account for most of these injuries, with falls being the predominant cause in the young and old, and motor vehicle collisions the primary source in young adults.[1] Addressing these mechanisms is a key component of public health prevention initiatives. In recent years, the cumulative effects of repeat mild TBI has gained attention with evidence suggesting the potential for delayed, trauma-related dementia; as a result, in 2010 the National Football League established 5 centers of excellence in the United States dedicated to cognitive assessments for retired players.[2]

Historically the designation "mild" TBI connoted a minimal risk of significant injury and implied the patient was at little or no risk for sequelae. However, using only a GCS may be misleading to both the patient and the clinician in that some patients with "mild" injury harbor a life-threatening intracranial lesion and other patients with "mild" injury develop delayed and/or persistent symptoms. Approximately 10% of patients with head trauma evaluated in the ED with a GCS score of 15 will have an acute lesion on head computed tomography (CT), however, fewer than 1% of these patients will require neurosurgical intervention.[3-5] Depending on how disability is defined, up to 15% of patients with mild TBI will have compromised function 1 year after their injury.[6,7] The objective in the initial evaluation of these patients is to determine who has an acute traumatic intracranial injury and who can be safely discharged from the acute care setting. A second challenge, which has not been met, is to identify those patients at risk for having postconcussive symptoms. There are at least 3 practice guidelines that have been written to help in the assessment and discharge planning of adults and children who have sustained a TBI.[8-10]

Department of Emergency Medicine, Mount Sinai School of Medicine, One Gustave L. Levy Place, Box 1620, New York, NY 10029, USA
E-mail address: andy.jagoda@mssm.edu

Psychiatr Clin N Am 33 (2010) 797–806
doi:10.1016/j.psc.2010.09.004
0193-953X/10/$ – see front matter © 2010 Elsevier Inc. All rights reserved.

MILD TBI CLINICAL ASSESSMENT

There is no consensus definition of mild TBI. Mild TBI may not be clinically evident during the initial evaluation, due to symptom resolution or the employment of insensitive assessments. Head injury is defined as clinically evident trauma above the clavicles, such as lacerations, ecchymosis, and forehead abrasions, but does not necessarily include TBI: TBI refers to an injury of the brain itself, and may manifest either as lesions on neuroimaging or as subtle changes on neuropsychological examinations. Concussion is a term that is used interchangeably with mild TBI and defined in various ways in the literature, often in the context of sports injuries.

Initially developed to describe patients in coma after head injury, the GCS is the most widely used tool for reporting global brain function after trauma (**Table 1**).[11] A score of 13 to 15 is typically classified as mild; however, a single GCS score is irrelevant and must be placed in the context of serial evaluations. A low GCS that remains low or a high GCS that decreases predicts a poorer outcome than a high GCS score that remains high or a low GCS score that improves. In one of the original multicenter studies validating the scale, approximately 10% of patients who became comatose had an initial GCS of 15.[12]

The Centers for Disease Control and Prevention (CDC) has developed a conceptual definition for mild TBI[13]: occurrence of injury to the head, resulting from blunt trauma or acceleration or deceleration forces, with one or more of the following conditions attributable to the head injury during the surveillance period:

1. Any period of observed or self-reported transient confusion, disorientation, or impaired consciousness
2. Any period of observed or self-reported dysfunction of memory (amnesia) around the time of injury
3. Observed signs of other neurological or neuropsychological dysfunction
4. Any period of observed or self-reported loss of consciousness lasting 30 minutes or less.

History and physical examination in the ED have proved to be insensitive for predicting which patients will develop sequelae. Consequently, in recent years research has

Table 1
Glasgow Coma Scale: score of 13–15 = mild; 9–12 = moderate; less than 9 = severe

Criterion	Adult	Score
Eye opening	Spontaneous	4
	To speech	3
	To pain	2
	None	1
Motor response	Obeys	6
	Localizes	5
	Withdraws	4
	Abnormal flexion	3
	Extension	2
	None	1
Verbal response	Oriented	5
	Confused	4
	Inappropriate	3
	Incomprehensible	2
	None	1

attempted to identify more sensitive measures including biomarkers, advanced bedside neurocognitive testing, and diagnostic instruments for assessing attention. At the present time there is no conclusive evidence supporting the routine use of any of these modalities; however, research is promising.

Biomarkers

Biomarkers play an important role in detecting and monitoring many disease processes, perhaps most notably myocardial infarction. Proteins and molecules have been identified that are released after a brain injury, cross the blood-brain barrier, and reach the peripheral circulation where they can be quantified in laboratory assays. Several brain-specific neuronal and astrocyte proteins have been studied for their ability to predict traumatic abnormalities identified on head CT after mild TBI. The best studied biomarker to date is S100B. S100B rises and falls rapidly after mild TBI with an approximate serum half-life of 97 minutes; measurement must be made within 4 hours of the injury.[8] At a cutoff of 0.10 µg/L the sensitivity approaches 100%. Studies have reported sensitivities of 90% to 100%, but low specificities of 4% to 65%, in predicting acute traumatic lesions on head CT.[14–16] As of 2010, no biomarker has been approved by the Federal Drug Administration; however, a practice guideline codeveloped by the CDC and the American College for Emergency Physicians (ACEP) identifies a potential future role and gives a weak level of recommendation to the consideration of using S100B as a screen to decide which patients are candidates for neuroimaging.[8]

Computerized Neurocognitive Testing

Patented software is currently available for bedside testing of 4 neurocognitive domains: verbal memory, visual memory, visual motor speed, and reaction time. This battery of tests can be administered at the bedside using a laptop computer. Preliminary, ED-based studies suggest that these batteries may identify subtle deficits in patients with isolated mild TBI; however, no correlation with outcomes has been reported. These studies report impairments in visual motor speed and reaction time without statistically appreciable verbal or visual memory score deficits.[17]

Devices for Assessing Attention

Focusing on the mechanism of injury in mild TBI, researchers have suggested that the shearing of connections in the frontal area of the brain results in deficits in attention and memory. Building on this postulate that there is a correlation between deficits in attention and abnormalities in smooth-pursuit eye movement, the Brain Trauma Foundation has developed a device that assesses eye tracking, which can be done quickly (in <1 minute). Preliminary tests suggest that this eye-tracking device is highly accurate, and clinical trials are currently being performed.[18]

RADIOLOGICAL IMAGING

Radiological imaging in the acute evaluation of the patient with mild TBI centers on 2 nodal decision points: who needs to be imaged and what is the most appropriate imaging modality, that is, plain skull films, head CT, or magnetic resonance imaging (MRI).

Skull Radiographs

The literature is conclusive that skull radiographs are neither sensitive nor specific for detection of intracranial injury after head trauma. A meta-analysis published in 2000 examined the association between skull fracture and brain injury, and reported that they are neither sensitive nor specific for identifying intracranial lesions.[19] A skull fracture increases the probability of an intracranial lesion fivefold; however, its low sensitivity precludes its use to rule out the diagnosis of an intracranial traumatic lesion and thus is of limited clinical value in risk stratification for brain injury. Current guidelines do not recommend plain film radiographs in the evaluation of patients with mild TBI.[8]

Noncontrast CT

Trauma registries reflect that approximately 10% of patients with mild TBI have an acute traumatic injury on noncontrast head CT, though only approximately 1% of these patients have a lesion requiring a neurosurgical intervention.[3–5] The literature does not provide a clear association of positive CT and the development of postconcussive symptoms, nor is it clear from the literature which patients with minor asymptomatic acute traumatic lesions (eg, smear subdural hemorrhage, traumatic subarachnoid hemorrhage) progress and ultimately require neurosurgical interventions. Most practice guidelines and decision rules have focused on identifying any acute traumatic lesion as the primary outcome measure and not just those that require neurosurgical intervention.

The 2 most commonly referenced decision rules for determining which patients with a mild TBI need a CT scan are the New Orleans Criteria (NOC)[3] and the Canadian CT Head Rule (CCHR)[4]; both have been validated prospectively (**Table 2**). In the CCHR, the investigators concluded that CT in mild TBI is indicated only in those patients with 1 of 5 high-risk factors: failure to reach a GCS score of 15 within 2 hours of injury, suspected open skull fracture, sign of basal skull fracture, vomiting more than once, or age older than 64 years. The NOC are the result of a derivation study that was then validated prospectively and identified 7 predictors of abnormal CT scan findings: headache (any head pain), vomiting, age older than 60 years, intoxication, deficit in short-term memory (persistent anterograde amnesia), physical evidence of trauma

Table 2
Criteria for determining if CT is indicated after minor head injury CT is Needed if the Patient Meets One or More of the Following Criteria (see text for explanation of these 2 rules/criteria)

New Orleans Criteria: Mild TBI with GCS = 15	Canadian CT Head Rule: Mild TBI with GCS = 13–15
Headache	High risk (for neurosurgical intervention):
Vomiting	GCS score <15 at 2 h after injury
Age older than 60 years	Suspected open or depressed skull fracture
Drug or alcohol intoxication	Any sign of basal skull fracture
Persistent anterograde amnesia (deficits in short-term memory)	Vomiting >1 episode
Visible trauma above the clavicle	Age >64 y
Seizure	Medium risk (for brain injury on CT):
	Amnesia before impact >30 min
	Dangerous mechanism (pedestrian struck by motor vehicle, occupant ejected from motor vehicle, fall from height >3 ft or 5 stairs)

above the clavicle, and seizure. Absence of all 7 findings had a negative predictive value of 100% (95%; confidence interval 99%–100%).

The presence of any of the clinical elements in the NOC and the CCHR criteria essentially identify all patients requiring emergent neurosurgical intervention. Both rules have low specificity; Canadian rule use would result in a 37% reduction in CT scans whereas the New Orleans Rule would reduce CT scans by only 3% to 20%. The difference in specificity is attributable to the CCHR's primary outcome measure being a neurosurgical lesion whereas the NOC's primary outcome measure is any acute traumatic intracranial lesion.

Studies that provided external validation of the NOC and CCHR have identified several limitations of these rules.[20,21] Both decision rules use loss of consciousness or amnesia as entry criteria, and neither applies to patients on anticoagulants. Therefore, neither rule can be reliably applied to all patients with head trauma. In addition, if the primary outcome measure of acute traumatic lesion is used (without subcategorizing into significant and nonsignificant as done in the CCHR), it becomes clear that specificity is sacrificed for sensitivity. Consequently, clinicians are faced with the dilemma of choosing the outcome measure they are most interested in and deciding on the risk one is willing to take in missing an acute, nonsurgical lesion.

Data from several large databases identify clinical variables to consider when deciding on whether to image the mild TBI patient.[20,21] At the present time there is no good evidence that antiplatelet medications increase the chance of an intracranial lesion. Although identified in the NOC, neither seizure nor mild or moderate headache are significant univariate predictors of intracranial injury. Alcohol was also not found to be a univariate predictor of intracranial injury in these studies. A dangerous mechanism of injury does emerge as an important factor in deciding who requires neuroimaging.

Based on the best available evidence, the CDC/ACEP joint practice guideline on mild TBI makes 2 recommendations regarding who requires neuroimaging in the emergency department[8]: Based on high-quality evidence, that is, the New Orleans Study and subsequent validation studies, the guidelines make a "Level A" recommendation that a noncontrast head CT is indicated in head trauma patients with loss of consciousness or posttraumatic amnesia only if one or more of the following is present: headache, vomiting, age older than 60 years, drug or alcohol intoxication, deficits in short-term memory, physical evidence of trauma above the clavicle, posttraumatic seizure, GCS score less than 15, focal neurologic deficit, or coagulopathy. The guidelines make a "Level B" recommendation, that is, a moderately strong recommendation, that a noncontrast head CT should be considered in head trauma patients with no loss of consciousness or posttraumatic amnesia if there is a focal neurologic deficit, vomiting, severe headache, age 65 years or older, physical signs of a basilar skull fracture, GCS score less than 15, coagulopathy, or a dangerous mechanism of injury that includes ejection from a motor vehicle, a struck pedestrian, and a fall from a height of more than 3 ft (1 m) or 5 stairs.

MRI

There are currently no well-designed studies that evaluate the use of MRI within 24 hours of injury in mild TBI patients. Several other studies demonstrate MRI abnormalities that could be attributed to TBI including contusions, diffuse axonal lesions, and epidural hematomas.[22,23] However, none of these studies demonstrated obvious clinical relevance of abnormal MRI scans in patients with mild TBI, and none were conducted within an acute patient management and disposition time frame. Therefore, at this time no evidence-based recommendations can be made regarding the use of MRI compared with CT in the acute setting. As MRI technology continues to evolve and becomes more uniformly available, there could be a role for its future use in the acute evaluation of mild TBI.

DISCHARGE PLANNING FROM THE EMERGENCY DEPARTMENT

There are 2 components of planning discharge of patients who have sustained a mild TBI from the ED: assessment of safety, that is, risk of deterioration, and education regarding postconcussive symptoms, that is, post-TBI clinical course. Retrospective analyses of large databases support the safety of discharging most patients with a GCS of 15 and a normal CT.[24,25] Several caveats must be taken into consideration: most databases do not include patients who are on anticoagulants or who have had past neurosurgical procedures; many databases do not include patients who are on antiplatelet medications; and most controversial of all, most patients in large databases were imaged hours post injury, thus introducing the unanswered question of whether a patient might have been scanned too early to detect an evolving hemorrhage.

The literature supports the safe discharge of patients with a mild TBI who have a negative head CT. Perhaps the best study is a systematic review that encompassed more than 62,000 mild TBI patients who presented with a GCS of 15.[25] The investigators report that there were at most 11 cases in which the patient deteriorated after a normal CT; the retrospective nature of the review precluded an analysis to identify factors that may have contributed to the deterioration, for example, age or medications. The investigators concluded that the scientific evidence supports the use of head CT strategy to determine which mild TBI patients can be safely discharged. In a prospective study involving 1292 patients with a GCS of 15 and a negative CT, 3-month follow-up failed to identify any patient who deteriorated after discharge.[26]

The CDC/ACEP joint practice guideline on mild TBI recommends that "patients with an isolated mild TBI who have a negative head CT scan result are at minimal risk for developing an intracranial lesion and therefore may be safely discharged from the ED."[8] This recommendation does not apply to patients with a bleeding disorder, who are receiving anticoagulation therapy or antiplatelet therapy, or who have had a previous neurosurgical procedure.

Postconcussive Symptoms (PCS)/Neurobehavioral Sequelae

Fig. 1 provides recently developed discharge instructions for patients, which include the symptoms that are frequently reported by patients after a mild TBI. Postconcussive symptoms (PCS) are generally divided into 3 domains: somatic, cognitive, and affective. The symptoms usually extinguish over time and rarely persist longer than 6 months. However, symptoms are common in the immediate weeks after injury, being frequently reported in patents 1 month after the injury (see article in this issue "Neurobehavioral Sequelae" by Riggio and Peters). Consequently, education regarding PCS is a key component of discharge planning of a patient evaluated for mild TBI in the ED. There is limited research on discharge planning, although there is evidence to suggest that education about PCS may reduce long-term complaints.[27,28] The presence of headache, nausea, and dizziness during the acute head injury evaluation may be prognostic of developing PCS.[29] The relative contributions that physical injury, premorbid mental health, and socioeconomic factors have on developing PCS remain unknown. Most likely the development of PCS is a multifaceted process with varying contributions of the aforementioned factors, depending on the individual. Of note, in a classic study Rimel and colleagues[7] reported that ongoing litigation did not affect the

Hospital:

What to expect after a
concussion

A part of CDC's *"Heads Up"* Series

INFORMATION FOR ADULTS

You have been examined for a head injury and possible concussion.

You did not have a CT scan of your brain because it was determined that it was not needed at this time.

You had a CT scan of your brain and no injury was identified.

It is safe for you to go home, but you may still have had an injury to your brain or may experience symptoms. We suggest that you limit certain activities.

Take time off from work or school for _____ days or until you and your health care professional think you are able to return to your usual routine.

Further instructions from your health care professional:

_____
_____
_____
_____
_____
_____

When should I return to the hospital emergency department?

Sometimes serious problems develop after a head injury. Return immediately to the emergency department if you experience any of the following symptoms:

Repeated vomiting

Headache that gets worse and does not go away

Loss of consciousness or unable to stay awake during times you would normally be awake

Getting more confused, restless, or agitated

Convulsions or seizures

Difficulty walking or difficulty with balance

Weakness or numbness

Difficulty with your vision

Most of all, if you have any symptom that concerns you, your family members, or friends, **don't delay, see a doctor right away.**

Q&A. Some questions and answers about brain injuries

Q. What is a concussion?

A. A concussion is a type of traumatic brain injury (TBI). It is caused by a bump, blow, or jolt to the head or body that causes the head and brain to move quickly back and forth. Some of the ways you can get a concussion are when you hit your head during a fall, car crash, or sports injury. Health care professionals sometime refer to concussions as "mild" brain injuries because they are usually not life-threatening. Even so, their effects can be serious.

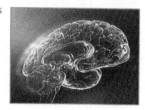

Q. What should I expect once I'm home from the hospital?

A. Most people with a concussion recover quickly and fully. During recovery, it is important to know that many people have a range of symptoms. Some symptoms may appear right away, while others may not be noticed for hours or even days after the injury. You may not realize you have problems until you try to do your usual activities again.

Please turn over.

 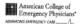 American College of Emergency Physicians®
ADVANCING EMERGENCY CARE

Fig. 1. Sample instructions developed by the Centers for Disease Control and the American College of Emergency physicians. These instructions are not copyrighted and can be downloaded at www.cdc.gov/concussion.

presence or absence of PCS; instead, socioeconomic support systems predicted return to work and persistence of symptoms. However, a systematic review of the literature including 9 studies did report a relationship between litigation and/or compensation issues with slower recovery after mild TBI.[30] It is estimated that patients with PCS miss on average 4.7 work days; up to 20% of patients with PCS are unemployed at 1 year.[31]

Recognizing the good possibility of a patient with mild TBI developing PCS, education is a key component of the discharge process. The CDC has collaborated with ACEP to develop sample discharge instructions that inform patients when to return to the ED, versus when to seek follow-up with a clinician experienced in sequelae of TBI (see **Fig. 1**). A key component of those discharge instructions includes information about PCS and recommendations on when to return to work/school/sports. One study using records from the National Hospital Ambulatory Medical Care Survey reported that 9% of mild TBI patients were discharged without any recommendations for follow-up and 28% had only "return to the ED as needed" as a follow-up recommendation.[32] In a review of discharge instructions from 15 institutions, Fung and colleagues[33] found only one institution had a discharge sheet that they considered complete (ie, contained 6 factors they deemed fundamental for safe monitoring). These investigators also found that most of the discharge instructions sheets were at an inappropriately high-grade reading level. There is literature to support the need for patients to receive both written and oral discharge instructions. In a small prospective study, Saunders and colleagues[34] found that mild TBI patients rarely remember their discharge instructions, which implies that it is best to provide discharge instructions in a written form after mild TBI. Levitt and colleagues[35] found that 23% of patients discharged from the ED with mild TBI could not remember any of their discharge instructions.

FUTURE DIRECTIONS

There remain many questions in need of study regarding mild TBI. Increased awareness of the neurobehavioral sequelae of mild TBI, cumulative effects of repeat injury, and chronic traumatic encephalopathy make the acute management of mild TBI key to maximizing good outcomes. First and foremost, there needs to be a better definition of what is "mild" TBI. The definition must incorporate the timing of the evaluation and the type of evaluation: single GCS scores are not predictive of outcome and the GCS is not sensitive enough to identify subtle dysfunctions. Standardization of the timing of the GCS determination, for example, in the field versus 1 hour post injury versus 3 hours post injury, would greatly facilitate research by defining similar populations and subsequent prognosis. Field testing is yet another important area in need of research: do field tests for attention and other parameters of neurological and/or psychological performance have a role risk stratifying patients and their outcomes? Timing of neuroimaging is a critical area in need of investigation and clarification for both categorization of injury and determination of outcome risk. Current recommendations are based on databases that include patients injured within 24 hours of presentation: rapid prehospital transport times and ready access to CT in the ED introduce the question of whether a patient can be scanned to detect an evolving lesion at an early stage. Neurodiagnostics in the form of biomarkers and neurocognitive evaluations in the ED in the postinjury period are yet other areas in need of investigation. Current evidence suggests that biomarkers may help to risk-stratify patients with a head injury and thus enable selective use of CT; this is of particular importance in children, for whom there is an imperative to minimize radiation exposure.

SUMMARY

The lack of uniformity in the definition of mild TBI, plus the absence of large, well-designed trials, makes interpretation of much of the mild TBI literature difficult at best. The dilemma that the acute care provider faces on a regular basis is which neurologically intact patients with mild TBI require a CT and who can be safely sent home, and when can they be sent home. Large databases have validated the NOC, which apply to TBI patients with a GCS of 15 who experienced trauma-related loss of consciousness or posttraumatic amnesia. Large databases have also revealed that neither loss of consciousness nor posttraumatic amnesia are discriminatory for identifying mild TBI patients at risk for harboring a neurosurgical lesion, thus making clinical decision making challenging. No set of clinical criteria has been established that identifies all patients with a neurosurgically significant lesion. There is a growing body of literature supporting the use of brain-specific biomarkers, and these markers may play an important role in the future in identifying patients requiring neuroimaging. All head-injured patients require education about their injury, with instructions on when and with whom to follow up.

REFERENCES

1. Rutland-Brown W, Langlois J, Thomas K, et al. Incidence of traumatic brain injury in the United States. J Head Trauma Rehabil 2006;21:544–8.
2. Available at: http://www.mercurynews.com/sports-headlines/ci_15626846?nclick_check=1. Accessed August 1, 2010.
3. Haydel MJ, Preston CA, Mills TJ, et al. Indications for computed tomography in patients with minor head injury. N Engl J Med 2000;343:100–5.
4. Stiell IG, Wells GA, Vandemheen K, et al. The Canadian CT head rule for patients with minor head injury. Lancet 2001;357:1391–6.
5. Smits M, Dippel D, de Haan G, et al. External validation of the Canadian CT head rule and the New Orleans criteria for CT scanning in patients with minor head injury. JAMA 2005;294:1519–25.
6. Alves W, Macciocchi S, Barth J. Postconcussive symptoms after uncomplicated mild head injury. J Head Trauma Rehabil 1993;8:48–59.
7. Rimel RW, Giordani B, Barth JT, et al. Disability caused by minor head injury. Neurosurgery 1981;9:221–8.
8. Jagoda AS, Cantrill SV, Wears RL, et al. Clinical policy: neuroimaging and decision making in adult mild traumatic brain injury in the acute setting. Ann Emerg Med 2002;40:231–49.
9. American Academy of Pediatrics. Management of minor closed head injury in children. Pediatrics 1999;104:1407–15.
10. Quality Standards Subcommittee of the American Academy of Neurology. Practice parameter: concussion in sports. Neurology 1997;48:581–5.
11. Teasdale G, Jennett B. Assessment of coma and impaired consciousness. A practical scale. Lancet 1974;2(7872):81–4.
12. Jennett B, Teasdale G, Galbraith S, et al. Severe head injuries in three countries. J Neurol Neurosurg Psychiatry 1977;40:291–8.
13. Centers for Disease Control and Prevention, National Center for Injury Prevention and Control. Report to Congress on mild traumatic brain injury in the United States: steps to prevent a serious public health problem. Atlanta (GA): Centers for Disease Control and Prevention; 2003. p. 1–47.
14. Bazarian JJ, Beck C, Blyth B, et al. Impact of creatine kinase correction on the predictive value of S-100B after mild traumatic brain injury. Restor Neurol Neurosci 2006;24:163–72.
15. Biberthaler P, Linsenmeier U, Pfeifer K-J, et al. Serum S-100B concentration provides additional information for the indication of computed tomography in patients after minor head injury. A prospective multicenter study. Shock 2006; 25:446–53.

16. Ingebrigtsen T, Romner B, Marup-Jensen S, et al. The clinical value of serum S-100 protein measurements in minor head injury: a Scandinavian multicentre study. Brain Inj 2000;14:1047–55.

17. Peterson S, Stull M, Collins M, et al. Neurocognitive function of emergency department patients with mild traumatic brain injury. Ann Emerg Med 2009;53: 796–803.

18. Maruta J, Suh M, Niogi S, et al. Visual tracking synchronization as a metric for concussion screening. J Head Trauma Rehabil 2010;25:293–305.

19. Hofman PAM, Nelemans P, Kemerink GJ, et al. Value of radiological diagnosis of skull fracture in the management of mild head injury: meta-analysis. J Neurol Neurosurg Psychiatry 2000;68:416–22.

20. Smits M, Diederik W, Dippel W, et al. Predicting intracranial traumatic findings on computed tomography in patients with minor head injury: the CHIP prediction rule. Ann Intern Med 2007;146:307 405.

21. Ibanez J, Arikan F, Pedraza S, et al. Reliability of clinical guidelines in the detection of patients at risk following mild head injury; results of a prospective study. J Neurosurg 2004;100:825–34.

22. Voller B, Benke T, Benedetto K, et al. Neuropsychological, MRI and EEG findings after very mild traumatic brain injury. Brain Inj 1999;13:821–7.

23. Hughes D, Jackson A, Mason D, et al. Abnormalities on magnetic resonance imaging seen acutely following mild traumatic brain injury. Neuroradiology 2004;46:550–8.

24. Livingston DH, Lavery RF, Passannante MR, et al. Emergency department discharge of patients with a negative cranial computed tomography scan after minimal head injury. Ann Surg 2000;232:126–32.

25. af Geijerstam JL, Britton M. Mild head injury: reliability of early head computed tomographic findings in triage for admission. Emerg Med J 2005;22:103–7.

26. af Geijerstam JL, Oredsson S, Britton M, et al. Medical outcome after immediate computed tomography or admission for observation in patients with mild head injury: randomised controlled trial. Br Med J 2006;333:465.

27. Andersson EE, Emanuelson I, Bjorklund R, et al. Mild traumatic brain injuries: the impact of early intervention on late sequelae. A randomized controlled trial. Acta Neurochir (Wien) 2007;149:151–60.

28. Ghaffar O, McCullagh S, Ouchterlony D, et al. Randomized treatment trial in mild traumatic brain injury. J Psychosom Res 2006;61:153–60.

29. Carroll I, Cassidy J, Peloso P, et al. Prognosis for mild traumatic brain injury: results of the WHO collaborating centre task force on mild traumatic brain injury. J Rehabil Med 2004;43(Suppl):84–105.

30. Binder L, Rohling M. Money matters: a meta-analytic review of the effects of financial incentives on recovery after closed-head injury. Am J Psychiatry 1996;153:7–10.

31. Dikmen SS, Temkin NR, Machamer JE, et al. Employment following traumatic head injuries. Arch Neurol 1994;51:177–86.

32. Bazarian JJ, McClung J, Cheng YT, et al. Emergency department management of mild traumatic brain injury in the USA. Emerg Med J 2005;22:473–7.

33. Fung M, Willer B, Moreland D, et al. A proposal for an evidenced-based emergency department discharge form for mild traumatic brain injury. Brain Inj 2006;20:889–94.

34. Saunders CE, Cota R, Barton CA. Reliability of home observation for victims of mild closed head injury. Ann Emerg Med 1986;15:160–3.

35. Levitt M, Sutton M, Goldman J, et al. Cognitive dysfunction in patients suffering minor head trauma. Am J Emerg Med 1994;12:172.

Traumatic Brain Injury and Its Neurobehavioral Sequelae

Silvana Riggio, MD[a,b,c,]*

KEYWORDS

- Traumatic brain injury • Postconcussive syndrome
- Neuropsychiatric disorders • Frontal lobe seizures

The development of neurobehavioral sequelae (NBS) associated with traumatic brain injury (TBI) is a multifactorial process. NBS is characterized by somatic and/or neuropsychiatric symptoms (**Box 1**). These clusters of symptoms have also been referred to in the literature as postconcussive symptoms or syndrome or disorder, but because these symptoms are not restricted to patients with concussion, but instead to TBI of all severities, the term, NBS of TBI, is more appropriate.

Evaluating TBI patients who present with neurobehavioral complaints requires a systematic history and physical that carefully defines the complaints and places them in the context of the injury, premorbid health, and postinjury circumstances. Somatic symptoms associated with NBS consist mostly of fatigue, lack of energy, sleep disturbances, dizziness, nausea, and headaches. Neuropsychiatric symptoms include cognitive and behavioral changes (ie, impairment of attention and/or memory, executive dysfunction, aggression, poor impulse control, irritability, anhedonia, or apathy). The complex of symptoms seen in TBI patients overlaps with several psychiatric disorders and/or neurological disorders or medical disorders. Complicating the presentation and diagnosis of TBI patients with suspected NBS are seizures. In particular, seizures of frontal lobe origin can be associated with bizarre behavioral manifestations and repetitive motor activity (RMA), which at times can be mistaken for a psychiatric manifestation.[1]

Evaluation of patients for NBS of TBI requires a structured history, including onset, duration, and severity of symptoms; environmental and social stressors; medical comorbidities; medications; and recreational drug use. It is key to delineate physiologic dysfunction and places deficits in the context of a patient's pre- and postinjury

[a] Department of Psychiatry, Mount Sinai School of Medicine, One Gustave L. Levy Place, Box 1230, New York, NY 10029, USA
[b] Department of Neurology, Mount Sinai School of Medicine, One Gustave L. Levy Place, Box 1230, New York, NY 10029, USA
[c] Department of Psychiatry, James J. Peters VAMC, 130 West Kingsbridge Road, Bronx, NY, USA
* Corresponding author. Department of Psychiatry, Mount Sinai School of Medicine, One Gustave L. Levy Place, Box 1230, New York, NY 10029.
E-mail address: silvana.riggio@mssm.edu

Psychiatr Clin N Am 33 (2010) 807–819
doi:10.1016/j.psc.2010.08.004
0193-953X/10/$ – see front matter. Published by Elsevier Inc.

psych.theclinics.com

Box 1
Neurobehavioral sequelae of traumatic brain injury

Neuropsychiatric

- Cognitive (eg, deficits in attention, memory, executive function)
- Behavioral[a]: aggression, irritability, poor impulse control, anhedonia, apathy, depressed mood, affective disorders
- Exacerbation of a primary psychiatric disorder (eg, affective disorders)
- Other

Somatic (eg, sleep disturbance, fatigue, dizziness, vertigo, headaches, visual disturbances, nausea, sensitivity to light and sound, hearing loss, seizures)

[a] Behavioral changes can be secondary to a primary psychiatric disorder versus possible underlying personality disorders and/or frontal/temporal lobe dysfunction or any central nervous system dysfunction secondary to the TBI.

---

psychiatric status. A careful physical examination is needed to establish the neurological baseline and identify deficits that may be contributing to the presenting complaint. For example, a subtle fourth or sixth cranial nerve injury (the most common neurological injuries in TBI patients) may contribute to headaches, difficulty concentrating, or sustaining attention. The physical examination must also include a comprehensive neurological and psychiatric mental status evaluation. It is only after a complete history and physical examination are performed that a clinician can decide which additional diagnostic studies are indicated (eg, neuroimaging, neurophysiologic, and/or neuropsychological testing).

The evolution or resolution of the symptoms over time is dependent on several variables, thus predicting the prognosis can be difficult.[2] Symptoms can vary, depending on the localization and lateralization of the injury, extent of the injury, medical and psychiatric comorbidities, and pre- and postpsychosocial factors. In addition, individual coping mechanisms play a significant role in recovery.

This article explores the NBS that may occur after TBI. A focus in this article is demonstrating the overlap of NBS with other conditions and providing a framework for developing a diagnostic and management strategy. The strategy must keep in mind both acute and long-term goals. Although pharmacotherapy is important in select cases, it can also be associated with side effects, which may interfere with a patient's function. Early rehabilitation, psychotherapy (eg, supportive, family, group, and behavioral) and cognitive rehabilitation are some of the measures that must be tailored to the individual.

CLINICAL OVERVIEW

Almost all TBI patients report some NBS in the acute phase after injury.[3] It is estimated that 30% to 80% of patients with mild to moderate TBI experience some NBS, which can persist for up to 3 months.[2] In adults, cognitive deficits are common in the acute stage, and the majority of studies indicate that in mild TBI complete recovery occurs within 3 to 12 months.[2] In up to 15% of mild TBI patients, NBS persist beyond 3 months and may contribute to long-term social and occupational difficulties; however, when this occurs, clinicians should aggressively look for contributing factors.[3–5] Cognitive dysfunction (eg, impaired attention, memory, and executive function) may play a predominant role in patients who experience persistent symptoms.[6] Identifying these deficits and developing an effective intervention plan may be critical to the successful recovery of patients. Risk factors for persisting symptoms, in addition to structural injury, include female gender, advanced age, pain, and prior affective or anxiety diagnoses.[7]

According to the World Health Organization Collaborating Center Task Force, a diagnosis of TBI-related NBS requires the presence of three or more of the following eight symptoms[2]:

- Headache
- Dizziness
- Fatigue
- Irritability
- Insomnia
- Concentration
- Memory difficulties
- Intolerance to stress, emotion, or alcohol

The overlap of NBS symptoms with primary affective disorders and cognitive disorders as well as other medical and neurological disorders makes differentiating the entities difficult. It takes a carefully designed evaluation to sort out these conditions. Factors that help distinguish one diagnosis from another include time of onset, duration of symptoms, and characteristics of the symptoms.

NEUROBEHAVIORAL SEQUELAE

Neurobehavioral sequelae consists of neuropsychiatric and somatic symptoms which can be present after a traumatic brain injury. The neuropsychiatric symptoms include cognitive and behavioral/psychiatric disorders.

NEUROPSYCHIATRIC SYMPTOMS
Cognitive Disorders

Cognitive complaints after TBI include impairment of attention/concentration, memory, and/or executive function.[8] There may be difficulties performing preinjury tasks and jobs or following instructions that would ordinarily be routine. Patients often report difficulty sustaining attention, planning, switching parameters, organizing, or sequencing, especially in the setting of a frontal lobe injury. These deficits may result in frustration and be expressed in the form of increased irritability, anxiety, apathy, or depression. Clinicians must determine if these symptoms are the result of the injury per se or a manifestation of the frustration of not performing at premorbid baseline.

The post-TBI evaluation of cognitive function must determine if performance problems are due to deficits in attention versus memory. If attention is impaired, there is difficulty retaining information with obvious impact on memory and thus performance. If a patient has an underlying affective disorder, attention can also be impaired due to lack of interest and/or distractibility. Therefore, the assessment of memory must be placed in context of attention and other disorders that may interfere with performance.

Persistence of cognitive deficits is related to some degree to severity of injury. In a systematic review of the literature, Dikmen and colleagues[8] reported that penetrating, moderate, and severe TBIs were associated with persisting cognitive deficits. Patients with mild TBI are a more difficult population to understand but the investigators concluded that there is insufficient evidence to associate mild TBI with persisting cognitive deficits past 6 months. Studies in the sports medicine literature demonstrate that cognitive deficits resulting from sports-related mild TBI generally resolve within days and rarely last more than 3 months.[9,10] These findings must be placed, however, in the context of patients who tend to be motivated and performance driven; these findings cannot necessarily be generalized to all subsets of patients who experience a mild TBI. Neither loss of consciousness nor posttraumatic amnesia (PTA) reliably stratifies those patients at greatest risk for cognitive deficits. The sports medicine literature on mild TBI has reported that cognitive impairments are most severe immediately after the closed head injury and resolved within 48 hours.[9,10] These findings support the importance of cognitive rest immediately after a mild TBI.

Behavioral/Psychiatric Symptoms

Behavioral disorders

There are several behavioral manifestations associated with TBI. Clinicians must determine if the symptoms were present before the injury or were the result of the injury (ie, primary cause or exacerbant). Behavioral manifestations can also be due to a primary psychiatric disorder that becomes expressed as a result of the stress of the injury. Weak defense mechanisms, poor social support, medications, and drug use can all complicate the presentation. Symptoms complex can also be complicated by an emotional response to the injury, its limitations, and fear of disability (**Fig. 1**).

Affective and behavioral disturbances after TBI may be expressed as personality changes appreciated by the patients or their family/caregiver. Personality changes may include aggression, impulsivity, irritability, emotional lability, or apathy.[11,12] These changes are more frequently reported after moderate and severe TBI; there is insufficient evidence linking many of these symptoms to mild TBI.[13] Impulsivity and irritability may lead to verbal and physical inappropriateness expressed as verbal outbursts or combativeness. They may be due to impaired judgment secondary to an underlying structural lesion or the exacerbation of an underlying psychiatric disorder or to an emotional response to trauma.

Depression

Major depression is one of the most frequently reported NBS of TBI; the actual prevalence varies from study to study based on methodology but seems to be approximately 25% to 50% after moderate to severe TBI versus a general population

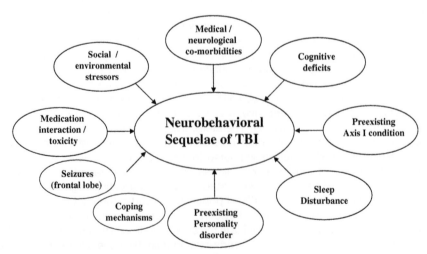

Fig. 1. Concomitant factors of NBS sequelae.

provalence of 17%.[14–16] The degree to which a premorbid psychiatric disorder increases the risk for NBS after TBI is unclear, but studies indicate a positive correlation: Seel and colleagues[17] described fatigue (29%), distractibility (28%), anger/irritability (28%), and rumination (25%) as the most common depressive symptoms in a prospective, multicenter study of 666 nonacute moderate to severe TBI patients. Twenty-seven per cent of the TBI patients met criteria for major depression, with feelings of hopelessness, worthlessness, and anhedonia differentiating depressed from nondepressed patients.

Risk factors for developing major depression after TBI fall into two categories: premorbid psychiatric pathology and low socioeconomic status. The relationship between rates of depression and the severity of TBI is unclear. The greatest chronicity of major depression, however, seems to occur in patients with both moderate to severe TBI and prior psychiatric illness.[2]

Studies have found a link between TBI and suicidality as well as between psychiatric comorbidity in the setting of TBI and suicidality.[18,19] In a retrospective study of 5034 patients, Silver and colleagues[18] reported that patients with a history of TBI with loss of consciousness had a 4-times greater likelihood of attempted suicide than those without TBI, 8.1% versus 1.9%. This risk of suicide attempt remained even after controlling for demographics, quality-of-life variables, alcohol abuse, and any comorbid psychiatric disorders. In a systematic review of the literature, Herdorffer and colleagues[10] found insufficient evidence linking mild TBI and completed suicide.

Anxiety disorders/Posttraumatic stress disorder

Anxiety disorders are reported after mild TBI, most commonly in individuals who also have a limb injury.[10,16] Increased age, a history of posttraumatic stress disorder (PTSD), and an avoidant coping style increase risk of acute stress symptoms after TBI.[20,21] An acute stress disorder predisposes to the development of PTSD after TBI: PTSD has been associated primarily with mild TBI in the military population whereas there is insufficient evidence linking it to mild TBI in the civilian population.[21]

Recall of a traumatic event has been identified as a predictor of developing PTSD.[22,23] Turnbull and colleagues,[23] in a study of 55 patients, reported that having traumatic memories of an injury were associated with increased psychological distress. Amnesia for events, although not protective against PTSD, was related to a decreased severity of symptoms. Other predictors of the development of PTSD, as well as its severity, include avoidant coping style, behavioral coping style (versus cognitive coping style), and prior unemployment (an indicator of premorbid level of functioning).[24] There is ongoing controversy regarding the relationship between PTSD and PTA, the point being the likelihood of having the disorder if a patient does not recall the traumatic event. The primary question is how patients can have PTSD if they cannot re-experience the actual trauma via intrusive thoughts or nightmares. The proposed counterargument in the controversy is the theory that TBI patients with PTA for a traumatic event re-experience the trauma event through the imagination from secondhand accounts or the patient's own mind[25] and that patients may also be able to re-experience fragments or islands of memory within the amnestic period, thus meeting the re-experiencing criterion of PTSD.[26]

The military experience does differ from the civilian experience regarding the association of PTSD with mild TBI: Hoge and colleagues[27] studied soldiers with mild TBI and a variety of postinjury symptoms. After adjusting for PTSD and depression, mild TBI was no longer significantly associated with symptoms except headache. The investigators postulated that PTSD and depression are important mediators of the relationship between mild TBI and physical health problems.

Aggression

Aggression is a commonly reported behavioral symptom of TBI, again, most commonly associated with moderate and severe injuries. Tateno and colleagues[8] studied 89 consecutive inpatients with moderate to severe TBI and found that 34% exhibited aggressive behavior within the first 6 months of injury. Risk factors for aggression after TBI include frontal lobe injury, premorbid affective disorder, personality disorder, or alcohol or substance abuse.

Substance related disorders

A review of the literature by van Reekum and colleagues[15] reported a 22% prevalence of substance abuse in TBI patients versus a 15% lifetime prevalence in the general population. A review of subsequent studies by Rogers and Read[14] in 2007 showed a prevalence of 12%. Premorbid substance use has been found to be strongly associated with post-TBI drug use, and many studies have cited substance abuse as a risk factor for TBI rather than vice versa. A 30-year longitudinal study by Koponen and colleagues[28] showed that 71% of TBI patients who were using drugs currently also did so pre-TBI. A systematic review of the literature found limited evidence of an association between TBI and decreased drug and alcohol use up to 3 years post injury.[10]

Somatic Symptoms

Headache

Headache is the most commonly reported somatic symptom after mild TBI with a prevalence ranging from 25% to 90%.[29–31] Post-TBI headaches may be classified as acute, beginning within 2 weeks of the injury and resolving within 2 months, or as chronic, beginning within 2 weeks and persisting for more than 8 weeks. The common co-occurrence of headache with other NBS was reported by Baandrup and Jensen.[30] Fifty-three per cent had at least one other somatic complaint (fatigability, sleep disturbance, dizziness, or alcohol intolerance), 49% had at least one cognitive complaint (memory dysfunction or impaired concentration/attention), 26% had at least one psychiatric complaint (irritability, aggressiveness, anxiety, depression, or emotional lability), 17% had all three types of complaints, and 17% had none.

A premorbid history of headache increases the risk of posttraumatic headaches, and those with pretraumatic headache may experience a worsening of the headache after injury. The presence of posttraumatic headache has not been consistently correlated with the severity of the injury; some investigators have reported that mild TBI patients have higher rates of headache during the initial posttraumatic phase than patients with more severe injury.[32] In the majority of mild TBI cases, headaches resolve within 3 months.[2]

Dizziness/Nausea

Dizziness is commonly reported after head injury although most studies do not separate the vague complaint of dizziness from that of vertigo.[33] The mechanisms of vertigo and dizziness are different and must be teased apart in the history and physical examination. Vertigo can result from a central or peripheral lesion with central lesions potentially being life threatening. In the acute phase, clinicians must always consider a vertebral artery dissection in TBI patients complaining of vertigo. Peripheral causes include cupulolithiasis, perilymphatic fistula, posttraumatic Meniere disease, damage to the vestibular nerve, and use of ototoxic medications. Dizziness/vertigo is reported in 24% to 78% of mild TBI patients acutely, significantly higher than the prevalence in non-TBI patients in the community.[34] As with headache, dizziness generally resolves within 3 months in patients with mild TBI whereas persistence may be more problematic in patients with moderate and severe TBI.[35] Anticholinergics (eg, meclizine) should be used judiciously, if at all, in treating patients with a complaint of dizziness; there is no good evidence to support their use and their sedative properties often make patients feel worse.

Fatigue

Fatigue is reported in up to 73% of patients post TBI and may become a persistent and debilitating symptom.[36–38] The presence of fatigue is associated with poorer social integration, decreased level of productive activities, and decreased overall quality of life. When fatigue persists, it may present a barrier to recovery. Post-TBI fatigue is most likely the result of a combination of causes, including pain, sleep disorders, cognitive deficits, depression, and anxiety. Hypopituitarism, with resultant neuroendocrine abnormalities, such as growth hormone deficiency and cortisol deficiency, may also be associated with post-TBI fatigue.[39] Other possible contributing factors include vertigo, diplopia, and iatrogenic causes, such as psychotropic or analgesic medications.

Sleep disturbance

Sleep disturbances are frequent after a TBI although the etiology is complex. These disturbances span the spectrum of sleep disorders and are reported in up to 73% of post-TBI patients.[40] Key to managing sleep disorders is identifying the factors contributing to the presentation.[41]

Seizures

Posttraumatic seizures can be focal or generalized; focal seizures can be simple or complex based on the lack (simple) or presence (complex) of loss of awareness or consciousness. Both simple and complex partial seizures can evolve into a secondary generalized seizure with tonic-clonic activity and postictal confusion. Due to the high incidence of TBI to the frontal or temporal lobe, the focus of posttraumatic seizures is often in these areas. Seizures of frontal lobe origin can be difficult to diagnose because they can present with a wide variety of clinical manifestations, frequently mimicking psychiatric disorders, yet can have a normal electroencephalogram (EEG).[1]

Seizures of frontal origin are often characterized by bizarre clinical manifestations, such as RMA, simple or complex automatisms (trashing, kicking, tapping, running, or agitation), and/or nonspecific auras, including dizziness or lightheadedness.[1] The bizarreness of frontal lobe seizures, without associated tonic-clonic activity or loss of consciousness, results in the diagnosis frequently being overlooked. To compound this issue, much of the frontal lobe is inaccessible to standard scalp EEG recording; consequently, the EEG can be normal even during an ictal episode. This can result in the false exclusion of a seizure disorder when too much reliance is placed on a single diagnostic test. Standard EEG in any type of focal epilepsy detects interictal epileptiform abnormalities in only 29% to 55% of patients and several series have reported no ictal EEG change in 33% to 36% of patients.[42] Some series have reported that only 14% of patients with frontal lobe seizures have localized frontal lobe discharges.[1]

Table 1 reviews some of the clinical characteristics of frontal lobe origin. When agitation, brief outbursts of rage and aggression, and/or new-onset bizarre behavior occurs in association with a TBI, a detailed history and careful characterization of the events are warranted. If the episodes are periodic, stereotypic, and brief in duration with a variable postictal phase, then the possibility of a frontal lobe seizure should be entertained.

Table 1
Clinical characteristics of frontal lobe seizures

Presentation	Frontal Lobe Seizure
Stereotypicity	Yes
RMA	Yes
Aura	Nonspecific
Duration	Brief
Abrupt onset	Yes
Abrupt ending	Yes
Postictal phase	Possible
Frequency	Often in clusters
Nocturnal	Possible
Situational	No
Goal directed aggression	No

Approach to Patients with Neurobehavioral Complaints After a TBI

Evaluating the NBS of TBI requires a deep understanding of a patient's neurological, psychiatric, and primary illness both pre- and post injury. At times, it can be difficult to differentiate NBS after a TBI from similar symptomatology secondary to a pre-existent psychiatric disorder. To complicate matters, affective symptoms can be the first clinical presentation of frontal lobe dysfunction independent of its origin and/or of a dementing process, possibly secondary to past TBIs (ie, chronic traumatic encephalopathy).

NBS are easier to put in context in patients with moderate or severe TBI who have demonstrable lesions on neuroimaging. The mild TBI group is more of a challenge and although the literature suggests the majority of patients make a complete recovery, there is a subset that does not.[2] Several studies have been performed trying to delineate the etiology and establish the existence of NBS in mild TBI; findings have been controversial and inconclusive.[2]

As discussed previously, the literature reports a high incidence of depression, anxiety, sleep disturbances, headaches/pain syndrome, fatigue, and dizziness in TBI patients. Many of these studies are underpowered, retrospective, or flawed by bias, however. In addition, most of the studies included patients of all TBI severities and included patients with prior psychiatric and substance abuse histories.[16] Studies of patients with pain and non–TBI-related injures report a high incidence of neurobehavioral complaints. A correlation between pain and NBS has been reported, and pain has been associated with the persistence of symptoms.[43–45] Occurrence of cognitive complaints in non-TBI chronic pain patients has been demonstrated, questioning the relationship between TBI per se and NBS.[45] Iverson and McCracken reported that non-TBI patients have a similar incidence of NBS as those patients with TBI.[43] They reported disturbed sleep, fatigue, and/or irritability in 81% of patients and one or more cognitive problems in 42% of patients.

Depression can be used as an example to demonstrate the difficulty linking NBS symptoms with TBI. To meet criteria for depression, five symptoms need to be present during a 2-week period: depressed mood and/or lack of interest plus insomnia, hypersomnia, fatigue or loss of energy, diminished ability to think or concentrate, and others. Some of these symptoms are commonly reported as NBS, however; depression due to TBI might be differentiated from a premorbid depression based on the onset of the symptoms associated presence of feeling worthlessness or hopelessness, significant weight changes, excessive guilt, or suicidal ideation. Bombardier and colleagues studied a cohort of 559 TBI patients and reported that 53.1% of the patients were depressed at some time within the 12 month after a TBI. The diagnosis was made after phone interview. Patients with prior history of depression or depression at injury were included. The study was conducted at a single level 1 trauma center and a high number of participants were Medicaid recipients. All of these factors might potentially have skewed the results.[16] They did not discuss the fact that depressed mood can be an NBS of TBI in the absence of other criteria. The same is true of fatigue, decrease in energy, decrease concentration, and sleep disturbances. All of these symptoms need to be considered in the setting of the injury, the individual response, past and present comorbidities, and concomitant pharmacotherapy.

In adjustment disorder, the development of emotional or behavioral symptoms occurs in response to an identifiable stressor. Predominant symptoms are depressed and anxious mood, which can occur individually or can be mixed depending of the subtype. Disturbance of conduct that is manifested by behavioral changes can also be present, in which case both the affective and the behavioral components can be misinterpreted with NBS. Symptoms usually occur within 3 month of the onset of head trauma, which is similar to what happens in NBS.

The major question confronting clinicians is whether or not outcomes change when patients are treated with antidepressants for depressed mood or anxious mood even if these symptoms are not secondary to major depression but are in the context of the psychosocial stressors often encountered after a TBI. There is insufficient evidence to answer this question, and future studies must try to determine the relative contributions of central nervous system lesions, physical disabilities, and environmental stressors on the manifestation of NBS. The importance of answering this question is obvious: There are risks of pharmacotherapy especially when a patient is cognitively compromised after a TBI. Antidepressants can interfere with cognitive function, especially with attention and memory, and can cause sleep disturbances. Also, headaches and extrapyramidal movements can be associated with antidepressant therapy and potentially interfere with motor function, especially in the elderly, or in patients in whom motor function is already compromised from the injury.

DIFFERENTIAL DIAGNOSIS AND MANAGEMENT PLAN

Determining the origin of a neurobehavioral complaint requires a systematic and comprehensive evaluation. NBS of TBI are nonspecific and clinicians must be careful to not draw a false conclusion before a proper assessment has been made. For example, TBI patients with a depressed mood may have a major depressive disorder but could also have an adjustment disorder, a lesion in the mesial frontal region, injury to the basal ganglia, or hypothyroidism. An adjustment disorder might not require pharmacotherapy whereas a major depression disorder does; depression from a mesial frontal lesion would have questionable benefit from antidepressants. Depression from a basal ganglia lesion could potentially get worse with antidepressants due to the possibility of secondary extrapyrimadal symptoms with bradykinesia mimicking psychomotor retardation. Not only must the cause of the depression be determined but also clinicians must remember the possibly the depression may be an expression of an existing condition and not directly due to the TBI.

Cognitive deficit of attention plays a major role in NBS and recognizing them may be the key to a successful management plan. The differential diagnosis of dysfunction of attention includes structural lesions, an underlying medical problem, a primary

---

Box 2
Frontal lobe lesions and its clinical presentations

Dorsolateral frontal region: Injury may be expressed as difficulties in switching parameters or planning; a certain mental inflexibility can be noted, which can ultimately result in irritability, slowness in performance, and/or low frustration tolerance, with potential social and performance repercussion.

Orbitofrontal region: Injury can manifest clinically with agitation, disinhibition, and/or poor impulse control.

Medial frontal region: Injury can manifest itself with apathy, which can be misdiagnosed with major depression.

---

psychiatric disorder, or drug side effect (in particular, compounds with high anticholinergic properties or antihistaminergic properties). Sleep disturbances and pain syndromes can also interfere with attention. Attention can be affected by a lesion in the orbitofrontal region, resulting in high distractibility, or due to a lesion in the dorsolateral region, resulting in an inability to switch mindset or to multitask (**Box 2**). Mood disorder, anxiety disorder, psychotic disorder, and/or personality disorder can also interfere with attention, as can fatigue secondary to the injury or to a medical problem.

Bizarre or unusual behavior after TBI can be the result of structural lesions, psychiatric disorders, drug toxicity, metabolic disorders, or frontal lobe seizures. Frontal lobe seizures deserve special mention because their clinical presentation can be characterized by bizarre behavior (eg, RMA), or automatisms, such as repetitive tapping, kicking, running, or trashing. These episodes can be associated either with or without loss of awareness, no loss of consciousness, nonspecific auras, and variable postictal confusion (see **Table 1**). Findings can appear psychiatric in origin and presentation can be associated with a normal interictal or ictal EEG.[1]

Complaints of NBS after TBI are best addressed by a multidisciplinary team. Family involvement is important to promote an understanding and support system needed for successful management. The literature on mild TBI demonstrates that education can decrease the severity and duration of NBS, partially by normalizing the situation and providing the reassurance needed to patiently allow recovery to occur.[4] Ponsford and colleagues[4] studied 202 mild TBI patients and reported that patients given an information booklet on mild TBI and coping strategies for symptoms were significantly less symptomatic at 3 months than those who were not provided education. An extensive review of articles on early intervention after mild TBI by Borg and colleagues[46] showed that early educational information reduce long-term complaints.

SUMMARY

The development of NBS after TBI is associated with several factors, making the identification of cause and the prognosis challenging. The severity of symptoms has some relation to the severity of injury. NBS after mild TBI are difficult to diagnose and treat because neuroimaging and physical examination are often normal. When present, NBS after mild TBI generally resolve within 3 months and when they become more persistent, a search for contributing factors beyond the initial injury should be done. To accomplish this, a systematic and comprehensive evaluation should be performed and the presenting complaint must be placed in the context of a patient's premorbid state. Neuroimaging is generally nondiagnostic in patients with mild TBI and NBS; thus, additional assessment may require neurophysiological and neuropsychological testing. Treatment of patients with TBI and NBS cannot be accomplished without a clear understanding of the underlying cause and the treatment must be placed within a patient's social and functional framework. Normalizing the experience through education to patients and their families facilitates recovery.

REFERENCES

1. Riggio S, Harner RN. Repetitive motor activity in frontal lobe epilepsy. In: Jasper H, Riggio S, Goldman-Rakic PS, editors. Epilepsy and the frontal anatomy of the frontal lobe. New York (NY): Raven Press; 1995. p. 153–66.
2. Carroll LJ, Cassidy JD, Peloso PM, et al. Prognosis for mild traumatic brain injury: results of the WHO collaborating centre task force on mild traumatic brain injury. J Rehabil Med 2004;(Suppl 43):84–105.
3. Alves W, Macciocchi S, Barth J. Postconcussive symptoms after uncomplicated mild head injury. J Head Trauma Rehabil 1993;8:48–59.
4. Ponsford J, Willmott C, Rothwell A. Impact of early intervention on outcome following mild head injury in adults. J Neurol Neurosurg Psychiatry 2002;73: 330–2.
5. Ruff RM, Camenzuli L, Mueller J. Miserable minority: emotional risk factors that influence the outcome of a mild traumatic brain injury. Brain Inj 1996;8:61–5.
6. Lundin A, de Boussard C, Edman G, et al. Symptoms and disability until 3 months after mild TBI. Brain Inj 2006;20:799–806.
7. Meares S, Shores EA, Taylor AJ, et al. Mild traumatic brain injury does not predict acute postconcussion syndrome. J Neurol Neurosurg Psychiatry 2008;79:300–6.
8. Dikmen S, Corrigan J, Levin H, et al. Cognitive outcome following traumatic brain injury. J Head Trauma Rehabil 2009;24:430–8.
9. Bleiberg J, Cernich AN, Cameron K, et al. Duration of cognitive impairment after sports concussion. Neurosurgery 2004;54:1073–80.
10. McCrea M, Guskiewicz KM, Marshall SW, et al. Acute effects and recovery time following concussion in collegiate football players: the NCAA concussion study. J Am Med Assoc 2003;290:2556–63.
11. Tateno A, Jorge RE, Robinson RG. Clinical correlates of aggressive behavior after traumatic brain injury. J Neuropsychiatry Clin Neurosci 2003;15:155–60.
12. Greve KW, Sherwin E, Stanford MS, et al. Personality and neurocognitive correlates of impulsive aggression in long-term survivors of severe traumatic brain injury. Brain Inj 2001;15:255–62.
13. Hesdorffer D, Rauch S, Tamminga C. Long term psychiatric outcomes following traumatic brain injury: a review of the literature. J Head Trauma Rehabil 2009; 24:452–9.
14. Rogers JM, Read CA. Psychiatric comorbidity following traumatic brain injury. Brain Inj 2007;21:1321–33.
15. van Reekum R, Cohen T, Wong J. Can traumatic brain injury cause psychiatric disorders? J Neuropsychiatry Clin Neurosci 2000;12:316–27.
16. Bombardier CH, Fann JR, Dikmen SS, et al. Rates of major depressive disorder and clinical outcomes following traumatic brain injury. JAMA 2010;303:1938–45.
17. Seel RT, Kreutzer JS, Rosenthal M, et al. Depression after traumatic brain injury: a national institute on disability and rehabilitation research model systems multi-center investigation. Arch Phys Med Rehabil 2003;84:177–84.
18. Silver JM, Kramer R, Greenwald S, et al. The association between head injuries and psychiatric disorders: findings from the new haven NIMH epidemiologic catchment area study. Brain Inj 2001;15:935–45.

19. Simpson G, Tate R. Suicidality in people surviving a traumatic brain injury: prevalence, risk factors and implications for clinical management. Brain Inj 2007;21: 1335–51.
20. Bryant RA. Posttraumatic stress disorder and traumatic brain injury: can they coexist? Clin Psychol Rev 2001;21:931–45.
21. Harvey AG, Bryant RA. Predictors of acute stress following mild traumatic brain injury. Brain Inj 1998;12:147–54.
22. Gil S, Caspi Y, Ben-Ari IZ, et al. Does memory of a traumatic event increase the risk of posttraumatic stress disorder in patients with traumatic brain injury? A prospective study. Am J Psychiatry 2005;162:963–9.
23. Turnbull SJ, Campbell EA, Swann IJ. Post-traumatic stress disorder symptoms following a head injury: does amnesia for the event Influence the development of symptoms? Brain Inj 2001;15:775–85.
24. Bryant RA, Marosszeky JE, Crooks J, et al. Coping style and post-traumatic stress disorder following severe traumatic brain injury. Brain Inj 1999;14: 175–80.
25. Bryant RA, Harvey AG. Relationship between acute stress disorder and posttraumatic stress disorder following mild traumatic brain injury. Am J Psychiatry 1998; 155:625–9.
26. King NS. Post-traumatic stress disorder and head injury as a dual diagnosis: "Islands" of memory as a mechanism. J Neurol Neurosurg Psychiatry 1997;62: 82–4.
27. Hoge CW, McGurk D, Thomas JL, et al. Mild traumatic brain injury in soldiers returning from Iraq. N Engl J Med 2008;358:453–63.
28. Koponen S, Taiminen T, Portin R. Axis I and II psychiatric disorders after traumatic brain injury: a 30-year follow-up study. Am J Psychiatry 2002;159:1315–21.
29. Uomoto JM, Esselman PC. Traumatic brain injury and chronic pain: differential types and rates by head injury severity. Arch Phys Med Rehabil 1993;74:61–4.
30. Baandrup L, Jensen R. Chronic post-traumatic headache—a clinical analysis in relation to the international headache classification 2nd edition. Cephalgia 2005;25:132–8.
31. Paniak C, Reynolds S, Phillips K, et al. Patient complaints within 1 month of mild traumatic brain injury: a controlled study. Arch Clin Neuropsychol 2002;17:319.
32. Couch JR, Bearss C. Chronic daily headache in the posttrauma syndrome: relation to the extent of head injury. Headache 2001;41:559.
33. Chamelian L, Feinstein A. Outcome after mild to moderate traumatic brain injury: the role of dizziness. Arch Phys Med Rehabil 2004;85:1662–6.
34. Anstey KJ, Butterworth P, Jorm AF, et al. A population survey found an association between self-reports of traumatic brain injury and increased psychiatric symptoms. J Clin Epidemiol 2004;57:1202–9.
35. Masson F, Maurette P, Salmi LR, et al. Prevalence of impairments 5 years after a head injury, and their relationship with disabilities and outcome. Brain Inj 1996;10:487–97.
36. Bushnik T, Englander J, Wright J. The experience of fatigue in the first 2 years after moderate-to-severe traumatic brain injury: a preliminary report. J Head Trauma Rehabil 2008;23:17–24.
37. Cantor JB, Ashman T, Gordon W, et al. Fatigue after traumatic brain injury and its impact on participation and quality of life. J Head Trauma Rehabil 2008;23:41–51.
38. Ashman TA, Cantor JB, Gordon WA, et al. Objective measurement of fatigue following traumatic brain injury. J Head Trauma Rehabil 2008;23:33–40.

39. Popovic V. Growth hormone deficiency as the most common pituitary defect after TBI: clinical implications. Pituitary 2005;8:239–43.
40. Rao V, Rollings P. Sleep disturbances following traumatic brain injury. Curr Treat Options Neurol 2002;4:77–87.
41. Clinchot DM, Bogner J, Mysiw WJ, et al. Defining sleep disturbance after brain injury. Am J Phys Med Rehabil 1998;77:291–5.
42. Quesney LF. Seizures of frontal lobe origin. In: Pedley T, Meldrum B, editors, Recent advances in epilepsy, vol. 3. London: Churchill Livingstone; 1986. p. 81–100.
43. Iverson GL, McCracken LM. 'Postconcussive' symptoms in persons with chronic pain. Brain Inj 1997;11:783–90.
44. Hart RP, Martelli MF, Zasler ND. Chronic pain and neuropsychological functioning. Neuropsychol Rev 2000;10:131–49.
45. McCracken LM, Iverson GL. Predicting complaints of impaired cognitive functioning in patients with chronic pain. J Pain Symptom Manage 2001;21:392–6.
46. Borg J, Holm L, Peloso PM, et al. Non-surgical intervention and cost for mild traumatic brain injury: results of the WHO collaborating centre task force on mild traumatic brain injury. J Rehabil Med 2004;43(Suppl):76–83.

Head Computed Tomography Interpretation in Trauma: A Primer

Joshua Seth Broder, MD

KEYWORDS

• Head • Computed tomography • Trauma • Interpretation
• Brain • CT • Diagnosis

Traumatic head injuries are a common cause of morbidity and mortality. Noncontrast computed tomography (CT) is the most common imaging modality used to evaluate these injuries in the emergency department. This article discusses key CT interpretation skills and reviews important traumatic brain injuries that can be discerned on head CT. It focuses on imaging findings that may deserve immediate surgical intervention. In addition, the article reviews the limits of noncontrast CT and discusses some advanced imaging modalities that may reveal subtle injury patterns not seen with CT scan.

HEAD CT ACQUISITION

Modern CT scanners can acquire a noncontrast head CT in less than 10 seconds. Typically, the patient is positioned in a supine position on the CT table and passes through the CT gantry headfirst. Modern CT scanners are equipped with multiple x-ray detectors, commonly numbering between 16 and 64, although CT scanners with more than 256 detectors are available. X-rays are emitted from a tube on one side of a circular gantry, pass through the patient, and strike the array of detectors on the opposite side. The gantry housing the x-ray tube and detectors is in constant circular motion. During the CT scan, the table holding the patient passes rapidly through the circular gantry. The combination of the circular motion of the gantry and the perpendicular linear motion of the patient results in a helical pattern of three-dimensional image data acquisition. From this data set, planar images can be reconstructed in the axial, sagittal, or coronal planes. For trauma evaluation, axial images are most commonly viewed. Modern CT scanners have the ability to acquire collimated radiographic data at a slice thickness of less than 1 mm. A typical adult human head is approximately 15 to 20 cm (150–200 mm) from skull base to vertex, so display of 1-mm slices would result in 150 to 200 images per head CT. Pragmatically, this is an

Division of Emergency Medicine, Department of Surgery, Duke University Medical Center, Box 3096, 2301 Erwin Road, Durham, NC 27710, USA
E-mail address: joshua.broder@duke.edu

Psychiatr Clin N Am 33 (2010) 821–854
doi:10.1016/j.psc.2010.08.006
0193-953X/10/$ – see front matter © 2010 Elsevier Inc. All rights reserved.

excessive number of images to review, and most important traumatic conditions do not require this resolution. Consequently, the original image data is typically reconstructed as a series of 5 to 10 mm thick slices for review. The typical head CT therefore consists of approximately 30 image slices.

With the patient positioned supine in the CT scanner and facing directly forward, the brain is tilted within the calvarium with the anterior portion of the brain tipped cephalad relative to the posterior portion. The CT gantry is tilted to match the brain orientation, allowing true perpendicular slices to be acquired (**Fig. 1**).

INTRODUCTION TO HEAD CT INTERPRETATION

To interpret a head CT scan, certain basic facts must be appreciated about the appearance of tissues and the orientation of a head CT scan. Modern CT scanners can acquire three-dimensional volumes of image data as described earlier. However, most noncontrast head CT scans are displayed and reviewed as a series of consecutive image slices in the axial plane. By convention, a slice is displayed with the patient's right-hand side on the left-hand side of the image. The anterior portion of the patient's head and brain is located at the superior aspect of the image (**Fig. 2**). The point of view of the observer is as if standing at the foot of the supine patient, looking toward the patient's head.

THE HOUNSFIELD CT DENSITY SCALE

CT was independently invented by the British physicist Sir Godfrey Hounsfield and the American Allan Cormack. Hounsfield's name has remained associated with the CT density scale, which is measured in Hounsfield units (HU).[1] The zero value on the scale

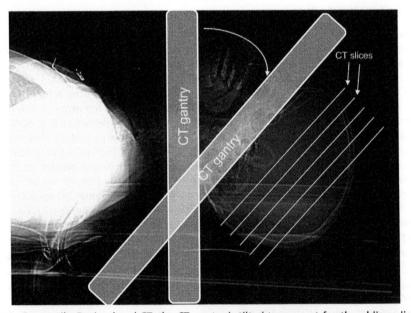

Fig. 1. Gantry tilt. During head CT, the CT gantry is tilted to account for the oblique lie of the brain within the calvarium, rather than being positioned perpendicular to the patient table. This position produces CT slices that section the brain in an anatomically relevant fashion, rather than crossing through multiple different levels of the brain.

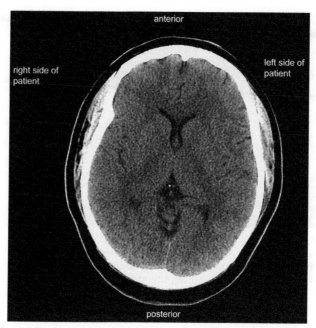

Fig. 2. Orientation of CT images. By convention, axial head CT slices are displayed with the anterior portion of the head at the top of the image and the posterior portion of the head at the bottom of the image. The right side of the patient is displayed on the left side of the image and the left side of the patient is displayed on the right side of the image. The perspective of the viewer is as if positioned at the patient's feet, looking up toward the head.

is arbitrarily set to the density of water. Air is given a value of −1000 HU. Dense bone is given a value of +1000 HU. The density of tissues measured with CT depends on their attenuation of the x-ray beam, which is proportional to their physical density. Fat is denser than air, but less dense than water, with a density of approximately −50 HU. Other soft tissues, including brain tissue, contain substantial amounts of water and are slightly denser than water, approximately +40 HU. Blood has a density higher than that of water because of its cell and protein content; the density and CT appearance of blood depend on its hematocrit and whether the blood has clotted. Acute clotted intracranial blood usually appears hyperdense to brain (bright white) with a density greater than +60 HU, whereas hyperacute blood may be hypodense (darker than both brain and clotted blood), with several theories postulated for this low density.[2–4] **Fig. 3** shows the CT appearance and Hounsfield densities of various tissues. The subtle differences in tissue densities can be used diagnostically, as discussed later in this article. Brain white matter contains myelin, which is rich in fat. As a consequence, white matter has a lower density than gray matter, which has a lower fat content. Because tissues with low densities appear darker than tissues with higher densities on CT, white matter (fat containing, and less dense) appears gray, and gray matter (lower in fat, and denser) appears white (**Box 1**).

CT WINDOWS AND TISSUE APPEARANCES

In a CT image, the density of tissues is depicted with a grayscale. The least dense tissues are assigned a black hue, and the highest density tissues are assigned pure

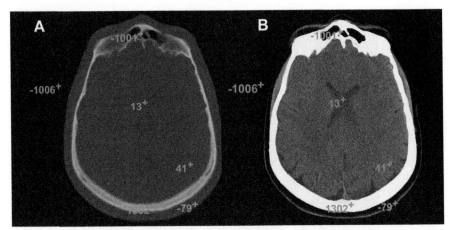

Fig. 3. Hounsfield density of tissues and window settings. (*A*) A CT image displayed using bone windows. (*B*) The same image data, displayed using brain windows. Windows allow the gray shades assigned to various densities to be adjusted to accentuate tissues of interest. The numerical values indicate the HU density at each cross-hair cursor location. Air has a density of −1000 HU, water 0 HU, fat approximately −50 HU, brain approximately +40 HU, and bone approximately +1000 HU.

white. Intermediate densities are assigned corresponding intermediate gray shades. The relative density of 2 tissues is fixed. However, the hue assigned to a given density can be varied to accentuate tissues of interest, a process called windowing. For example, rather than distributing all available gray shades across the full range of densities from air to bone, the hues can be distributed more narrowly within a given density range. All tissues less dense than the target range then appear completely black. All tissues more dense than the target range appear completely white.

Two windows settings are commonly used to evaluate head CT (see **Fig. 3**). A brain window broadly distributes the gray shades from the low density of air to the high density of bone. This window is useful for evaluation of hemorrhage, brain tissue, cerebrospinal fluid (CSF) spaces, and mass effect, as described in more detail later. Using a brain window, air appears black, adipose tissue nearly black, and CSF a very dark gray (nearly black). Air can be difficult to distinguish from adjacent low-density soft tissues on this window setting. Brain tissues appear as varying shades of gray depending on their water and fat content. Fresh blood appears a bright white, whereas subacute hemorrhage can vary in its density and typically appears a darker gray. Bone appears bright white, leading to a bloom artifact that can obscure fine lines of nondisplaced fractures.[5] For this reason, brain windows are not useful for identification of subtle fractures, as shown later in this article. Use of a bone window decreases bloom artifact.

Box 1
Gray matter and white matter
Pearl
When viewed with brain windows:
Gray matter (unmyelinated) appears whiter
White matter (myelinated) appears grayer

A bone window more narrowly distributes the gray shades across the high densities of bone. This distribution allows more subtle differentiation of the internal structure of bone including fractures. With a bone window, air appears black, soft tissues appear a dark gray, and bone appears a light gray approaching white in color. Consequently, bone windows are useful not only for delineation of subtle nondisplaced fractures but also for identification of pathological intracranial air, which is distinct in its appearance from adjacent low-density soft tissues on this window setting (**Figs. 4** and **5**). Bone windows are not useful for identification of brain parenchymal injury, intracranial hemorrhage, or CSF abnormalities, as these tissues share the same gray appearance on this window setting.

A window is defined by 2 values, a center value and a width. The center value is the Hounsfield density that is assigned the middle hue in the available gray shades. The width is the number of HU more than and less than the center value at which tissues are represented by absolute white and absolute black, respectively. A narrow width allows fine differentiation of density differences within a narrow range. However, all tissues less than the density range of the window appear completely black, and all those with densities greater than the window's width appear completely white, preventing differentiation of tissues outside of the window's range.

Many digital radiology viewing systems (called Picture Archiving and Communication Systems [PACS]) have preset drop menus allowing selection of the desired window. Window settings have not been fully standardized nationally, and in some cases it may be advantageous to alter the window setting subtly to improve visualization of structures. At the author's institution, a preset brain window has a center value of 42 HU and a width of 155 HU. However, narrowing the window to a center value

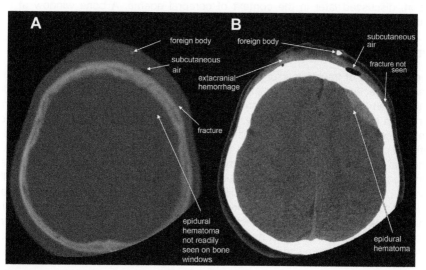

Fig. 4. Subcutaneous air, foreign bodies, and hemorrhage. (*A*) Bone windows. (*B*) The same image viewed with brain windows. Air in the subcutaneous tissues may be introduced through lacerations or adjacent sinus fractures. Air appears black on brain and bone windows. Note that fat and air have a similar appearance on brain windows. Subcutaneous foreign bodies may be visible on both brain and bone windows, depending on their density. Subcutaneous hemorrhage appears bright on brain windows. A systematic approach is needed to avoid missing pathology; this patient has intracranial hemorrhage (an epidural hematoma) as well as multiple extracranial findings. This is not seen on bone windows. Also notice that the fracture is visible using bone windows but not brain windows.

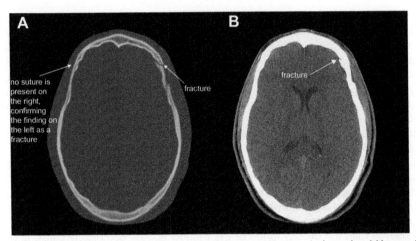

Fig. 5. Bone windows accentuate fractures. Both bone and brain windows should be used to identify all disorders on head CT. Nondisplaced fractures may be difficult or impossible to detect using brain windows. Here, a slightly displaced fracture is readily seen with bone windows (A) but is barely perceptible using brain windows (B). Compare with the previous figure, in which a nondisplaced fracture is invisible using brain windows. Always compare suspected fracture locations with the contralateral side to avoid mistaking a cranial suture for a fracture.

of 40 HU and a width of 80 HU can improve the visibility of gray-white matter differentiation, discussed later in the context of cerebral edema. A bone window at the author's institution has a center value of 570 HU and a width of 3077 HU (**Box 2**).

MIDLINE SHIFT AND MASS EFFECT

Specific forms of traumatic injury are discussed later in this article. More important than any specific injury is the presence of midline shift and mass effect. These abnormalities can indicate a need for immediate surgical intervention to prevent cerebral herniation and death. Consequently, every head CT interpretation must assess for their presence. Findings of midline shift and frank herniation on CT must be correlated with the patient's clinical examination. Rarely, patients with these findings may have a normal neurological examination. In the National Emergency X-radiography Utilization Study (NEXUS II) study of more than 28,000 adults, only 1 in 1500 neurologically normal patients had herniation or midline shift on CT. No neurological deficit was found in 1.9% of patients with CT findings of herniation and 4.4% of those with significant midline shift . However, all had other major brain abnormalities (including tumors and hemorrhage) accounting for mass effect and midline shift.[6] CT findings of herniation and midline shift are almost always clinically important, not incidental findings.

Box 2
Use of brain and bone windows

Pearls

Use bone windows to identify fractures and intracranial air

Use brain windows to identify hemorrhage, edema, midline shift/mass effect, loss of gray-white matter differentiation, and abnormalities of CSF spaces

Mass Effect

Mass effect refers to the deviation or distortion of normal structures by an abnormal structure or mass. In trauma, the pathological mass is most often hemorrhage, such as a subdural or epidural hematoma. Edematous brain matter and even foreign bodies may exert mass effect in some cases. Outside of trauma, neoplasms and infections may result in mass effect, although these are beyond the scope of this article. Recognition of mass effect requires some familiarity with the normal appearance of intracranial structures. The normal symmetry of the brain can aid the novice interpreter; asymmetry may indicate that one hemisphere is experiencing pathological mass effect. The structure experiencing mass effect may be a solid brain structure, or a fluid-filled compressible space such as a ventricle, cistern, or sulcus. Solid structures appear deviated from their normal position or deformed. Fluid-filled structures can be more subtle in their response to mass effect. For example, a ventricle may shift in location, or it may become completely compressed or effaced by increasing mass effect. The absence of a normal fluid-filled space should therefore be noted, because it may indicate significant mass effect.

Midline Shift

The brain is normally a symmetrical structure, and variations from this symmetry can indicate significant abnormalities. The midline of the brain is marked by the falx cerebri, a thin dural fold that forms a vertical sickle shape in the midsagittal plane in the longitudinal fissure separating the cerebral hemispheres. Symmetrically arrayed on either side of this line are brain structures including the caudate nucleus, thalamus, hypothalamus, internal capsule, and lentiform nucleus. The CSF-filled lateral ventricles are also symmetrically distributed to the right and left of the midline. Midline shift describes mass effect that results in movement of intracranial structures across the midsagittal line. Midline shift should be measured, because shift greater than 5 mm can lead to subfalcine herniation and death. In the presence of subdural or epidural hematoma, midline shift greater than 5 mm is an indication for acute neurosurgical evacuation to relieve mass effect, regardless of the patient's Glasgow Coma Score (current guideline from Brain Trauma Foundation, endorsed by the Congress of Neurological Surgeons).[7–10] On a digital PACS (a computer diagnostic imaging display), calipers allow ready measurement of midline shift. A line is drawn from the anterior midline calvarium to the posterior midline calvarium. The distance of deviation of the falx cerebri or other midline structures from this line is then measured (**Fig. 6**).

Pitfalls in CT Interpretation Related to Brain Symmetry

Some significant traumatic injuries can be present despite a symmetrical head CT scan. Bilateral subdural hematomas and parafalcine (midline) subdural hematomas can result in symmetry, as can diffuse subarachnoid hemorrhage. Narrow window settings can aid in detection of isodense subdural hematomas by allowing fine discrimination between similar densities in the narrow density range spanning blood and brain. Cerebral edema, hydrocephalus, and diffuse axonal injury (DAI) can be present despite a symmetrical brain CT scan. These injuries are discussed later in this article.[11]

ARTIFACTS AND NORMAL VARIATIONS SIMULATING DISEASE

Several common artifacts and normal variations may confuse the novice interpreter of brain CT. Although the brain is normally symmetrical, the patient may be positioned asymmetrically in the CT scanner, artificially creating an asymmetrical appearance.

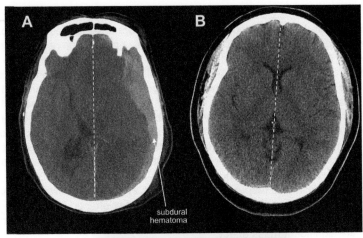

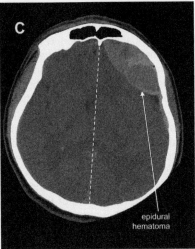

Fig. 6. Mass effect and midline shift. Mass effect and midline shift are critical findings on head CT, because significant midline shift indicates threatened or completed subfalcine herniation. The presence of midline shift may be more important than the specific type of injury that is the cause. (*A*) A large left subdural hematoma causing significant midline shift. (*B*) A normal brain with symmetrical distribution of structures about the midline. (*C*) A large left frontal epidural hematoma causing mass effect and slight midline shift. In each image, a dotted line has been added to accentuate the midline. The size of the brain lesion and the degree of midline shift should be measured and communicated to the neurosurgeon.

The interpreter must mentally compensate for asymmetry caused by patient positioning to avoid mistaking this for a disorder. Dense metallic objects within or outside the patient can create streak artifact, a star-burst appearance that can mask underlying abnormalities (**Fig. 7**). Dense bone in the occipital region can have a similar effect, making evaluation of the posterior fossa with CT poor compared with other brain regions. With advancing age, calcifications commonly occur in the choroid plexus in the bilateral posterior horns of the lateral ventricles, in the pineal gland in

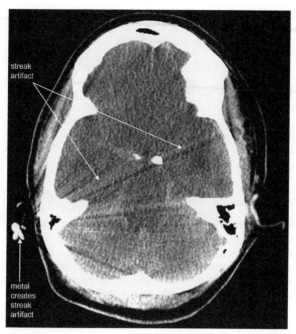

Fig. 7. Streak artifact. Dense material such as metal within or outside of the patient can create streak artifact that interferes with image interpretation. In this patient, extracranial metal creates streak artifact.

the midline, and in the basal ganglia. These calcifications can be mistaken for punctuate hemorrhage if the observer is not aware of the occurrence of these as a normal finding (**Fig. 8**).

A MNEMONIC FOR HEAD CT INTERPRETATION: ABBBC

A systematic approach to interpretation of head CT must be used to avoid a common error: stopping the interpretation prematurely after an obvious abnormality is detected. In 1998, Perron and colleagues[12] showed that use of the simple mnemonic BCBVB (blood can be very bad, for blood/cisterns/brain/ventricles/bone) improved emergency medicine resident accuracy in head CT interpretation and was retained for 3 months. Broder (2006) devised the following ABBBC mnemonic to assess for major forms of traumatic injury, including pathological air, which is not assessed by the former BCBVB mnemonic.[13]

A is for Air

Air is a normal finding within the sinus spaces of the skull, including the frontal, ethmoid, maxillary, and sphenoid sinuses. In addition, the mastoid processes normally contain air. These spaces normally do not contain fluid; in trauma, fluid within these air-filled spaces is likely blood and should trigger a search for fracture of the adjacent bone. The cranial vault does not normally contain air, so air within the calvarium is pathological and should prompt a search for an associated fracture. Subcutaneous tissues may also contain air introduced through skin lacerations or vented from sinuses through fractures.

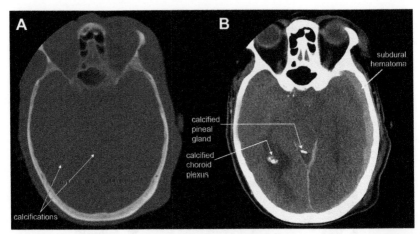

Fig. 8. Differentiating calcifications from blood. Calcifications commonly occur in the choroid plexus of the lateral ventricles and in the pineal gland. They may occasionally be found in other locations as well. Because both calcifications and blood appear bright on CT brain windows, calcifications may be mistaken for blood by novice CT interpreters. When in doubt, measure the HU. Blood has a Hounsfield density of approximately +50 HU, whereas calcified structures have densities generally greater than +500 HU. Bone windows may also help distinguish blood from calcifications. (*A, B*) The same image using bone and brain windows, respectively.

The search for air is best conducted using bone windows. Air appears black on both brain and bone windows, but bone windows accentuate this appearance, because no other tissue appears as dark. Using brain windows, air remains black but CSF and fat also appear dark and may interfere with detection of minute quantities of air. Using bone windows, fluid appears a moderate gray color.

Sinus air spaces
Inspection of the sinuses should be performed with attention to fluid levels within the sinus spaces. Because the patient is typically supine during the CT scan, fluid usually layers in dependent portions of the sinuses. In contrast, thickening of the sinus mucosa, which can occur because of sinusitis unrelated to trauma, is often circumferential and may or may not be associated with dependent fluid. Once an air-fluid level is detected within a sinus space, the surrounding bone should be inspected for fracture, as discussed later. The sinus may be completely filled with fluid, in which case no air-fluid level will be seen.

Mastoid air spaces
The mastoid air cells can also fill with fluid because of hemorrhage associated with temporal bone fracture. These air cells are minute (a few millimeters in size in an adult), so air-fluid levels are not seen. Instead, the black latticework of air within these spaces is replaced by fluid density, gray on CT bone windows. When this appearance is seen, a search for temporal bone fracture should be conducted. For both sinuses and the mastoid air cells, the contralateral side can provide a normal comparison, although bilateral injuries are possible.

Technically, fluid within these normally air-filled spaces cannot be identified as blood using CT. Preexisting mucous or purulent fluid has a similar density. As described earlier, circumferential mucosal thickening is more suggestive of preexisting sinus disease but, if no fracture is identified, even simple fluid may indicate fluid other than blood. In a patient without other signs or symptoms of sinus disease, the diagnosis of sinusitis should not automatically be made In response to CT findings, because studies have shown CT to be nonspecific for sinus infection, although some investigators dispute this.[14–16]

Figs. 9 and **10** compare normal and abnormal sinus air spaces.

Soft tissue air

Air within extracranial soft tissues can be introduced through external skin wounds or can escape from fractures of air-containing sinus spaces. On bone windows, air is black against the background of soft tissues, which appear an intermediate gray. If air is adjacent to sinus spaces, fractures of the walls of those spaces should be suspected and careful inspection should be performed. In addition, foreign bodies

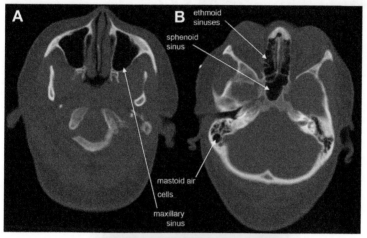

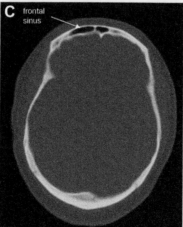

Fig. 9. (A, B, C) Normal sinus spaces. Facial sinuses should be inspected using bone windows. Normal sinuses are air-filled (black), with no evidence of fluid opacification (intermediate gray using bone windows). In trauma, fluid within sinuses may be blood related to adjacent fracture. When fluid is found within sinuses, inspect the walls of the sinus for discontinuity representing fracture. Compare these normal sinuses with the abnormal sinuses in the next figure.

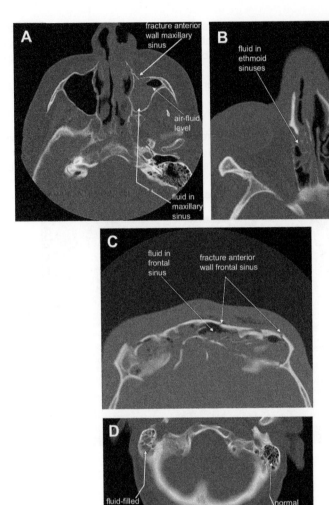

Fig. 10. Fluid in sinuses and mastoid air cells. In trauma, fluid in the normally air-filled facial sinuses and mastoid air cells can indicate blood from fractures. Compare these images with the prior figure. (*A*) A maxillary sinus fracture with fluid in the left maxillary sinus. (*B*) Fluid in ethmoid air cells. (*C*) A comminuted frontal sinus fracture with fluid in the frontal sinus. (*D*) Fluid in the right mastoid air cells.

resulting from wounds should be sought when subcutaneous air is found (**Fig. 11**, see **Fig. 4**).

Intracranial air

The cranial vault should be carefully inspected for air, which is never normally present in this location (**Fig. 12**). Air bubbles may be millimeters in size, or large collections of air may be seen. Fractures of the adjacent calvarium should be noted, and fractures of the posterior walls of the frontal and other facial sinuses should be sought. Air can also leak intracranially from a mastoid and associated temporal bone fracture.[17] Outside trauma, intracranial air can be a sign of infection with gas-forming organisms, as in

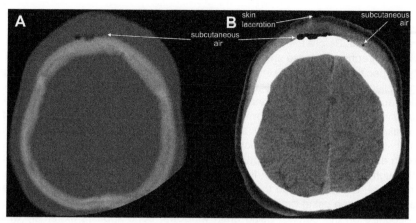

Fig. 11. Subcutaneous air. Subcutaneous air may be introduced from a skin laceration or a fracture of an adjacent sinus. Always inspect the adjacent bone for fractures and soft tissues for foreign bodies. (*A*) Bone windows. (*B*) Brain windows.

an intracranial abscess. Postoperative gas can be a normal finding in patients after craniotomy and may persist for weeks, with a half-life of approximately 1.5 days.[18] Rarely, air can be introduced iatrogenically through venous and arterial catheters.[19] Intracranial gas can also occur in dive-related decompression illness.

B is for Bone

The first "B" in our mnemonic stands for "bone." Numerous bony abnormalities may be seen on CT, including some unrelated to trauma, such as benign bone cysts and lytic lesions associated with malignancy. In trauma, the primary purpose of bone inspection is detection of fractures.

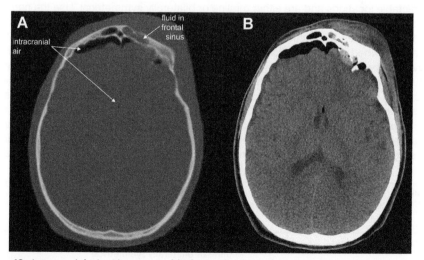

Fig. 12. Intracranial air. Air appears black on all CT window settings. However, on brain window settings, fat also appears nearly black. On bone windows, no other tissue appears black, making small amounts of air more conspicuous. This patient has a lot of intracranial air adjacent to the frontal sinus, caused by a fracture of the posterior plate of that sinus. (*A*) Bone windows. (*B*) Same image, brain windows.

Fractures

Fractures of bone may require little emergent treatment but nonetheless are a sign of significant force. Before the advent of CT, skull fractures were often diagnosed using skull radiographs, but these are no longer recommended because of a lack of sensitivity or specificity for the more important diagnosis, underlying brain injury. The American College of Emergency Physicians recommends against the use of skull radiographs in suspected mild traumatic brain injury.[20] The American College of Radiology gives skull radiographs its lowest appropriateness value (1 on a 9-point scale) for the evaluation of minor head injury, and 2 out of 9 for moderate or severe closed head injury.[21] One exception is in suspected child abuse, where skull radiographs are still used to document linear skull fractures, which may occasionally be missed with CT.

Although a major role of CT is to determine the presence of brain injury and hemorrhage, CT can be used to assess for skull and facial fracture. Displaced fractures can be seen using brain windows, but nondisplaced fractures can be difficult to recognize on this setting. Using brain windows, bone appears extremely white, and a bloom artifact occurs, which can disguise nondisplaced fractures. The preferred setting for evaluation of bony injury is the bone window, which renders dense cortical bone a less-bright white color. Fractures are visible as discontinuities in the bone.

Use of bone windows alone to view CT images rendered for assessment of brain does not provide the greatest possible bony detail, although it is likely sufficient for detection of most significant injuries. Other CT manipulations can be performed to improve bone evaluation. Image slices can be reconstructed at thinner slice thickness using the original CT image data (eg, 1-mm slices, rather than the 5-mm slices often used for brain assessment). In addition, the computer algorithm used to create the CT image from the original data can be altered. Bone reconstruction algorithms differ from soft tissue algorithms, although the details are beyond the scope of this article.

After selecting bone windows, inspect the entire calvarium for discontinuities that may represent fractures. Normal suture lines are visible as discontinuities but have predictable locations and are either midline or bilaterally symmetrical. Use the normal symmetry of the skull and knowledge of the expected locations of sutures to avoid mistaking sutures for fractures. When in doubt, inspect the surrounding tissues for air as described earlier, and, for hemorrhage, as described later. Soft tissue swelling may also be present overlying fractures but would not be expected with normal sutures. Vascular channels in bone may occasionally be mistaken for nondisplaced fractures, because these appear as lucencies within bone (**Table 1**). Like sutures, these should have no associated soft tissue air or underlying hemorrhage. Displaced fractures are typically readily apparent. Depression of fragments should be noted and measured, because depression of fragments greater than 5 mm is a relative indication for surgery to elevate fragments.[22] Intracranial air underlying a fracture can indicate

Table 1	
Differences among nondisplaced fractures, cranial sutures, and vascular channels	
Structure	**Features**
Cranial suture lines	Predictable location Midline or bilaterally symmetrical No associated intracranial hemorrhage or air
Vascular channels	No associated intracranial hemorrhage or air
Fractures	Often asymmetrical or unilateral May have associated intracranial air and hemorrhage

a dural tear and is an indication for surgical repair. Soft tissue defects and air overlying fractures should be noted, because a fracture underlying a laceration is an open fracture potentially benefiting from antibiotic prophylaxis. Some controversy exists about the role of antibiotics in this setting. A randomized trial showed no difference in the rate of meningitis in patients treated prophylactically with antibiotics and those receiving no antibiotics, but overall infectious complications were more common in the nonantibiotic group.[23] A Cochrane meta-analysis found no benefit to prophylactic antibiotics in basilar skull fractures.[24]

The absence of fractures does not rule out intracranial hemorrhage or other serious injury. Consequently, a complete assessment must be performed even if no fractures are identified. Some life-threatening brain injuries, including hemorrhage, edema, and DAI, may have no associated fractures. In children, the odds of intracranial hemorrhage in the presence of skull fracture are increased (odds ratio 2.17), but hemorrhage can occur in the absence of fracture.[25]

See **Figs. 4, 5** and **10**, which show facial and calvarial fractures.

Sinus inspection

As described earlier, fractures of facial sinuses and mastoid air cells may be suggested by the presence of abnormal fluid within these spaces. Inspect the sinuses for fluid and trace the bony perimeter of each space for discontinuities representing fractures.

B is for Blood

The second "B" in our mnemonic is for "blood," a key finding in traumatic injury. Several types of traumatic hemorrhage are possible, and recognition of the likely location of hemorrhage can have clinical importance, as described later (**Table 2**). The size or quantity of hemorrhage should be noted, and any associated midline shift or mass effect must be determined, because this may have greater clinical importance than the type of hemorrhage itself. The presence of active hemorrhage should be recognized, as described later. The search for blood should be conducted using CT brain windows.

Subarachnoid hemorrhage

Subarachnoid hemorrhage is bleeding into the subarachnoid space, the space between pia mater and arachnoid mater. The subarachnoid space includes the

Table 2
Differences in CT appearance among subarachnoid, subdural, epidural, intraparenchymal, and intraventricular hemorrhage

Hemorrhage Type	Features
Subarachnoid hemorrhage	Fills sulci, fissures, and cisterns
Subdural hematoma	Crescent shaped Does not cross midline Not restricted in anterior-posterior extent by cranial sutures
Epidural hematoma	Lens shaped (biconvex disc) May cross midline Restricted in anterior-posterior extent by cranial sutures
Intraparenchmyal hemorrhage	Varies in size from punctuate to very large Do not confuse with normal calcifications in choroid plexus, basal ganglia, and pineal gland
Intraventricular hemorrhage	Part of the subarachnoid space Can originate from any other form of bleeding Can be associated with development of hydrocephalus

spaces surrounding the gyri on the brain surface, the Sylvian fissure, and the ventricles and cisterns. These spaces are normally filled with CSF, which appears nearly black on brain windows. In the presence of subarachnoid hemorrhage, these spaces appear bright white (**Fig. 13**). Subarachnoid hemorrhage can be localized or diffuse. When diffuse, subarachnoid hemorrhage can fill the suprasellar cistern, giving this a bright starlike appearance (**Fig. 14**). The normal appearance of the cisterns is discussed later. Intravenous (IV) contrast is not necessary for detection of traumatic subarachnoid hemorrhage; if administered, IV contrast can obscure subarachnoid hemorrhage, because both appear white on brain CT windows.

In acute traumatic brain injury, head CT is likely extremely sensitive for detection of subarachnoid hemorrhage. Recent studies of CT in nontraumatic aneurysmal subarachnoid hemorrhage suggest sensitivities ranging between 91% and 100%.[26,27] Several factors may contribute to imperfect detection of subarachnoid hemorrhage. Minute quantities of blood may be difficult to detect. Blood with a low hematocrit may be less dense than blood with a normal hematocrit and may be less evident against the backdrop of CSF.[28] CT may become less sensitive with time, because of diffusion of blood away from its point of origin and changes in the oxidation state of hemoglobin.[29] These factors are of significant concern in suspected aneurismal hemorrhage, because the underlying aneurysm remains a potential threat if not addressed surgically or with endovascular embolization (coiling). In trauma, the danger of missing small quantities of blood is less clear. Most traumatic subarachnoid hemorrhage is self-limited and requires no specific therapy. For these reasons, and in contrast with common practice in suspected aneurismal subarachnoid hemorrhage, lumbar puncture is not usually performed in trauma to detect subarachnoid hemorrhage after a normal head CT. Delayed bleeding in patients with a normal CT is rare and repeated head CT following a normal CT is not routinely recommended, barring a change in the patient's symptoms or neurological status.[30] The possibility of aneurismal hemorrhage leading to the patient's trauma should always be considered, because the imperative to detect hemorrhage is then heightened.

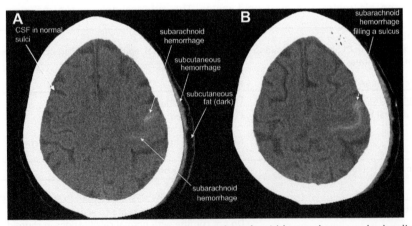

Fig. 13. Subarachnoid hemorrhage. Traumatic subarachnoid hemorrhage can be localized or diffuse. On brain windows, it appears bright and often follows the contours of cortical sulci, which are normally filled with dark CSF. Subcutaneous hemorrhage is also visible as a bright density beneath dark subcutaneous fat. (*A, B*) Adjacent axial CT slices, viewed with brain windows.

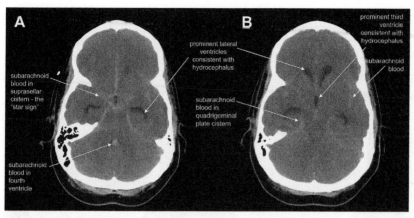

Fig. 14. Subarachnoid hemorrhage. Diffuse subarachnoid hemorrhage can escape notice because it can be a symmetrical abnormality. It may fill basilar cisterns and fissures. Subarachnoid hemorrhage can also block CSF reabsorption, leading to hydrocephalus, which is also visible in this case. Hydrocephalus is discussed later in this article. (*A, B*) Adjacent axial CT slices viewed with brain windows.

Blood in the subarachnoid space can obstruct the arachnoid granulations, which normally reabsorb CSF. The result can be communicating hydrocephalus, so CSF spaces should be carefully inspected for hydrocephalus when subarachnoid hemorrhage is identified. Evaluation of CSF spaces is discussed later.

Subdural hematoma

Subdural hematoma or hemorrhage is hemorrhage located in the subdural space, between the dura mater and brain surface. The appearance on CT brain windows is a variable gray color, depending on the age and acuity of hemorrhage. Acute subdural blood is usually hyperdense (brighter/whiter) to brain. As subdural blood ages, it can become isodense to brain (identical in color on CT) and eventually hypodense (darker) in appearance. Hemorrhage in the subdural space is usually caused by tears in small bridging veins from traumatic shear. Because the bleeding is venous, it is typically low pressure. Trapped between the dura and brain, the blood follows the brain contour and assumes a crescent shape, concave on its medial surface (**Fig. 15**; see also **Fig. 6**). Extension of the hematoma in anterior and posterior directions is not limited by the attachment points of the dura to the skull at suture lines, because the hemorrhage lies within the dural envelope. This distinguishes subdural hematoma from epidural hematoma, which is typically limited in its anterior-posterior extension by the attachment of the dura at cranial sutures. Rarely, epidural hematomas may cross suture lines because of crossing fractures or diastasis of sutures.[31] Each brain hemisphere is wrapped in its own dural layer. As a consequence, subdural hematomas do not usually cross the midline, although bilateral subdural hematomas are possible. Instead, on reaching the midline, a subdural hematoma may extend along the interhemispheric longitudinal fissure within the dura, following the medial surface of the hemisphere.

Although usually caused by low-pressure venous bleeding, subdural hematomas can become catastrophically large, leading to significant mass effect, midline shift, and herniation. The size of the subdural hematoma and any associated midline shift or mass effect should be carefully measured. According to current guidelines of the Brain Trauma Society and Congress of Neurological Surgeons, a subdural hematoma

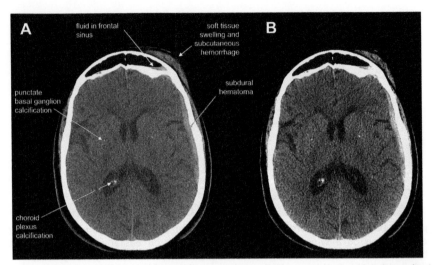

Fig. 15. Subdural hematoma. Subdural hemorrhage or hematoma appears bright on brain CT windows. The shape is characteristically a crescent with a concave medial surface, following the contour of the brain surface. Because the hemorrhage is contained within the dura mater, it is not restricted from anterior-posterior extension at cranial sutures, where the dura attaches to the calvarium. This patient has a small subdural hematoma with no appreciable midline shift. Compare with earlier figure on midline shift. (A, B) The same axial image, using slightly different brain window settings. Punctate calcifications are also seen in the basal ganglia bilaterally.

greater than 10 mm in thickness, or with greater than 5 mm of midline shift, is an indication for neurosurgical evacuation, regardless of the GCS of the patient.[7,10]

Subdural hematomas may experience recurrent hemorrhage, and the appearance can show blood of varying ages, as described earlier. A subdural hematoma containing multiple different gray shades indicates blood in various stages of decomposition, indicating multiple discrete episodes of bleeding. A mixed, swirling appearance of dark and bright shades with a subdural hematoma can indicate active bleeding (see **Fig. 6**).[32] Brighter densities within the hematoma are believed to represent clotted blood, whereas hypoattenuated regions (dark) are believed to represent unclotted blood from active hemorrhage.[33] This swirl sign, first described with epidural hematoma, should prompt rapid neurosurgical consultation, because an actively bleeding hematoma can also rapidly expand and may require surgical intervention.[34,35] Subacute or chronic subdural hematomas can be isodense with brain and may be extremely difficult to recognize (**Fig. 16**).[36] Acute subdural hematoma can be isodense with cortical gray matter in anemic patients.[3] A clue to the presence of an isodense subdural hematoma is the apparent absence of sulci on the affected side. The mass effect of the subdural hematoma may locally efface sulci at the brain surface, which may appear abnormally smooth compared with the crenelated appearance of the opposite normal hemisphere.

Epidural hematoma

An epidural hematoma is a collection of blood in the epidural space, between the external surface of the dura and the bone of the calvarium. The dura is typically attached to the skull at suture lines. Because an epidural hematoma expands to fill the space between the skull and the adherent dura, it assumes a biconvex disc shape,

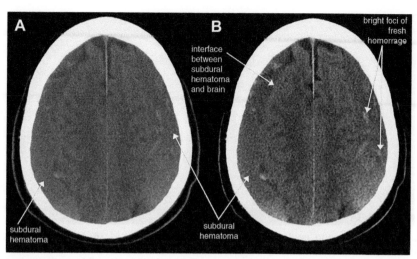

Fig. 16. Bilateral subdural hematomas. Subdural hematomas can be extremely subtle when bilateral. Rebleeding into subdural hematomas can occur. Fresher blood generally appears brighter. Older blood can become isodense with brain, making it difficult to recognize. Varying the window level slightly may make subdural blood more visible (*A* vs *B*, same image using slight variation in brain windows). This patient has large bilateral subdural hematomas with blood of varying ages. Note the absence of sulci because of their efface-ment by subdural blood. Midline shift is not seen here, because subdural hematomas are pushing the brain medially from both left and right.

in contrast with the crescent shape typical of subdural hematoma (**Figs. 17** and **18**; see also **Figs. 4** and **6**). The anterior-posterior extension of an epidural hematoma is usually restricted by the attachment of the dura at suture lines, unlike subdural hema-tomas, which can freely extend in an anteroposterior direction. In a study of pediatric patients, 11% of epidural hematomas crossed suture lines, so this feature alone cannot be used to distinguish subdural from epidural hematomas.[31] Unlike subdural hematomas, epidural hematomas can cross the midline. In the frontal region, an epidural hematoma may span the entire width of the frontal bone before being bounded bilaterally at the frontal sutures. In contrast, subdural hematomas reach the midline but do not cross, instead following the interhemispheric longitudinal fissure because of restriction within the dura mater.

Using CT brain windows, the appearance of an acute epidural hematoma is usually hyperdense (white) compared with adjacent brain. As with subdural hematomas, active bleeding may occur and is characterized by the swirl sign, a mixed heteroge-neous appearance of blood within the hematoma.

Classically, epidural hematomas are located in the temporoparietal region, are accompanied by temporal bone fracture (see **Figs. 17** and **18**), and result from injury to the middle meningeal artery. Because of their arterial source, they can rapidly expand, leading to herniation and death if not quickly evacuated surgically. The size of any epidural hematoma should be measured, as well as associated mass effect or midline shift. According to current guidelines of the Brain Trauma Foundation and Congress of Neurological Surgeons, an epidural hematoma greater than 30 cm^3 in volume (calculated using PACS tools) should be evacuated. Epidural hematomas less than 30 cm^3, with less than 15 mm thickness, or with less than 5 mm midline shift can be managed nonoperatively in patients with GCS greater than 8 and without focal

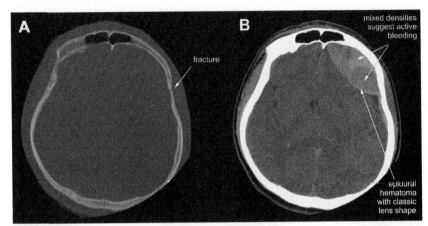

Fig. 17. Swirl sign and epidural hematoma. (*A*) Bone windows. (*B*) Same image, brain windows. This patient has a large epidural hematoma, with a classic biconvex disc (lens-shaped) appearance. On bone windows, an adjacent fracture is visible, a classic finding with epidural hematoma. The large epidural hematoma is creating mass effect and a small amount of midline shift is present. The mixed density of blood within the epidural hematoma has been called the swirl sign and is associated with active bleeding and rapid expansion. This patient, a 16-year-old boy, was alert on emergency department arrival but soon became unarousable. He underwent emergency craniotomy, was treated for a middle meningeal artery injury, and fully recovered.

neurological deficits. Anisocoria and GCS less than 9 are indications for surgery regardless of the size of the epidural hematoma.[8,9] Evidence of active bleeding has been correlated with fivefold increased mortality and (swirl sign, see **Fig. 17**) should also prompt rapid neurosurgical consultation and possible evacuation.[35] Other investigators have not found an association between the swirl sign and patient outcome.[4]

Intraparenchmyal hemorrhage
Like other forms of intracranial hemorrhage, intraparenchymal hemorrhage is best seen using brain windows. Acute intraparechymal hemorrhage appears hyperdense

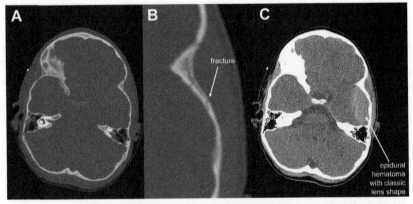

Fig. 18. Epidural hematoma. (*A*) Bone windows. (*B*) Close-up from (*A*). (*C*) Same image, brain windows. This patient has a classic epidural hematoma with a biconvex appearance and an associated temporal bone fracture. He underwent emergency craniotomy and recovered fully.

(white) relative to surrounding brain (**Fig. 19**). Unlike subdural and epidural hematomas, which lie on the brain surface, intraparenchymal hemorrhage occurs within the substance of the brain matter. The shape is usually rounded but may be amorphous and irregular. Intraparenchymal hemorrhage can extend into the ventricles. Hemorrhage of this type can be punctuate or large, with significant mass effect. It may be difficult in some patients to distinguish traumatic hemorrhage from spontaneous hypertensive hemorrhage or bleeding from an underlying lesion such as a malignancy or arteriovenous malformation. In some cases, CT angiography or other studies may be required to assess for an underlying lesion. The possibility of spontaneous hemorrhage leading to the patient's traumatic injuries should be entertained.

Multiple areas of punctuate intraparenchymal hemorrhage near the gray-white matter junction have been described as a finding associated with DAI, although axonal injury itself is not visible on CT.[37] DAI is discussed in more detail later.

Intraventricular hemorrhage

Intraventricular hemorrhage (**Fig. 20**) is bleeding within the ventricular system of the brain. The source is often subarachnoid or intraparenchymal hemorrhage. Acute blood within the ventricles appears white when using brain window settings, whereas normal CSF appears nearly black. Blood is denser than CSF and can form a fluid-fluid level within the ventricles, with dense blood in the dependent portions and less-dense CSF in nondependent regions. Patients are usually supine during medical care following trauma, including emergency medical services transport, emergency department care, and CT scan, so blood products may have sufficient time to layer in the ventricles by the time of the initial head CT.

Blood products within the ventricles can obstruct the reabsorption of CSF by arachnoid granulations, leading to hydrocephalus. When blood is seen within the ventricles,

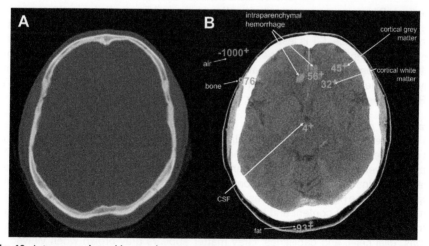

Fig. 19. Intraparenchymal hemorrhage. Intraparenchymal hemorrhage can vary in size from punctate to massive. This patient has bilateral frontal hemorrhages, sometimes referred to as contusions. These hemorrhages are nearly invisible on bone windows (*A*) but appear bright on brain windows (*B*). The density of blood is approximately +50 HU, denser than brain parenchyma (approximately 40–45 HU) but less dense than cranial bone (approximately +1000 HU). CSF is water density (approximately 0 HU). Air has a density of −1000 HU, and fat a density of approximately −50 HU. (*B*) Cursors have been placed to indicate the density of various tissues.

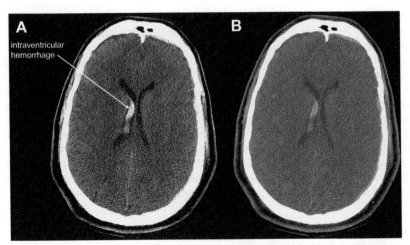

Fig. 20. Intraventricular blood. Intraventricular blood can arise from multiple sources, including primary subarachnoid hemorrhage, intraparenchymal hemorrhage, and subdural and epidural hematomas. The ventricles are contiguous with the subarachnoid space, and blood in this location can lead to hydrocephalus caused by obstruction of CSF reabsorption. (*A, B*) The same axial CT slice using slight variations in brain window settings.

the ventricles should be scrutinized for signs of hydrocephalus, which will be systematically assessed by our mnemonic regardless of the presence of blood.

B is for Brain

The final "B" in our mnemonic calls attention to "brain." Traumatic brain abnormalities are best assessed on CT scan using brain windows. Ironically, although injury to brain is of key importance, CT is less sensitive and specific for injury to the brain itself than for associated injuries such as hemorrhage and fractures. MRI provides exceptional soft tissue contrast, surpassing that achieved with CT, and can depict brain parenchymal injuries more directly, rather than relying on surrogate markers as with CT. MRI is discussed in more detail later.

Gray-white matter differentiation

As discussed earlier, the density of brain tissue depends on its composition, including fat and water content. The CT appearance depends in turn on the tissue density. White matter derives its name from the appearance of the tissue when viewed with the naked eye. It contains myelin-sheathed axons that are rich in fat, giving the tissue its white appearance. The high fat content results in a lower density compared with gray matter, which has lower fat content and higher water content than white matter. Gray matter contains a mixture of neuronal cell bodies, dendrites, myelinated and unmyelinated axons, glial cells, and capillaries. Gray matter appears gray-brown when viewed in an anatomic specimen.

The differences in density of gray and white matter contribute to differences in their CT appearance in both normal brain and injury or disease states. Normally, using CT brain windows, white matter appears darker than gray matter, because of its lower density. On a noncontrast head CT scan, normal gray matter structures can be differentiated from normal white matter structures (**Fig. 21**). Normal gray matter structures include the cortical gray matter, the caudate nucleus, the lentiform nucleus (containing

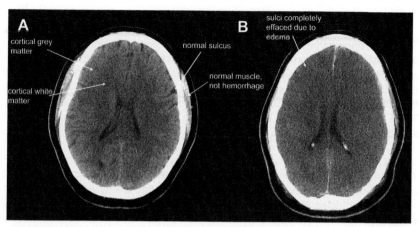

Fig. 21. Gray-white matter differentiation and cerebral edema. (*A*) A 26-year-old patient with normal brain with normal gray-white matter differentiation. (*B*) A 26-year-old patient with severe cerebral edema and loss of gray-white matter differentiation. This patient suffered brain death. Normally, a subtle difference in the appearance of gray and white matter is visible using CT brain windows because of differences in density, caused by the presence of myelin in white matter. Myelin contains low-density fat, which lowers the density of white matter relative to gray matter, making it darker on CT. In the presence of cerebral edema, the water content of brain tissues rises, making all brain tissues lower in density compared with their normal state. The subtle difference in density between gray and white matter is lost as a result. In addition, sulci become effaced by the increased volume of edematous brain.

the putamen and globus pallidus), and the thalamus and hypothalamus. Normal white matter structures include the cortical white matter and internal capsule.

Normal gray-white matter differentiation can be lost in traumatic injury. If focal brain ischemic and infarction occurs (familiar in nontraumatic ischemic stroke but also seen in traumatic injuries such as cervical arterial dissection with resulting embolic stroke), hypoperfused areas will be deprived of glucose and oxygen required for adenosine triphosphate (ATP) production. Without ATP, ATP-dependent cell membrane pumps, such as the sodium-potassium ATPase, will no longer function. Pump-dependent ion gradients will decay, and the distribution of water into tissues will follow these changes in ion gradients. As the water content of ischemic areas increases, their density will decrease relative to their normal values. These areas will become darker on the CT image. The border between gray and white matter will become indistinct because of localized edema. If the entire brain is affected by injury, diffuse cerebral edema may ensue, and global loss of gray-white matter differentiation may occur (see **Fig. 21**). As the brain swells, other findings of cerebral edema will become manifest in the adjacent CSF spaces (discussed later). If a local brain region is injured, local swelling of that structure may occur, and it may exert mass effect on adjacent intracranial structures, as discussed earlier.

C is for CSF Spaces

The final letter in our mnemonic is "C" for "CSF spaces." Normal intracranial spaces containing CSF include the sulci (the valleys separating the undulating gyri of the brain surface), fissures (deep invaginations in the brain, including the Sylvian fissure separating the parietal and frontal lobes superiorly from the temporal lobes inferiorly), cisterns (openings within the subarachnoid space, some large), and ventricles (including the lateral, third, and fourth ventricles). The relative size of these spaces is an important finding that can indicate the need for neurosurgical intervention, because it can reflect increases in intracranial pressure. The size of the brain in comparison with these CSF spaces must be noted and the patient's age should be incorporated into the evaluation. In addition, CSF spaces can be sites of intracranial hemorrhage including subarachnoid and intraventricular hemorrhage, discussed in detail earlier.

There are 4 important states of the brain, each with a distinct pattern of CSF spaces (**Table 3**, **Fig. 22**).

Normal CSF spaces

In the normal brain, in a young adult, the brain is well-developed and fills most of the calvarium. Some CSF does fill the sulci between gyri, and the Sylvian fissure is recognizable. The ventricles are open but not excessively large, and the cisterns, including the quadrigeminal cistern and suprasellar cistern, are visible. All contain CSF and appear nearly black on noncontrast CT using brain windows. The normal quadrigeminal cistern forms a smile-shaped black crescent, sometimes called the "smile sign" because it denotes a brain without evidence of significant edema or downward herniation. **Fig. 23** shows normal CSF spaces.

Cerebral atrophy

In cerebral atrophy (**Fig. 24**; see also **Fig. 22**), the entire brain appears small, and all CSF-containing spaces increase proportionally in size, because the intracranial volume is fixed. Sulci, fissures, ventricles, and cisterns all appear enlarged. In general, atrophy increases with increasing age. If an elderly patient's brain CT shows little sign of atrophy, this may indicate a healthy brain or an atrophic brain with superimposed diffuse edema (discussed later). Consequently, care must be taken to consider age and clinical condition when evaluating the CSF spaces.

Cerebral edema

In diffuse cerebral edema (**Fig. 25**; see also **Fig. 22**), the entire brain enlarges, at the expense of all CSF potential spaces, which decrease proportionally in size. Sulci, fissures, ventricles, and cisterns all become effaced. The normal smile sign of the quadrigeminal cistern is eliminated, a concerning finding that can indicate impending downward herniation. Several caveats bear mention in this evaluation. First, the patient's age should be taken into account. A young and healthy patient may have a well-developed brain without atrophy that nearly fills the calvarium, so a relative absence of sulci may be normal. However, normal ventricles and cisterns should not be slitlike or effaced. A patient with significant baseline atrophy may have significant superimposed edema before true effacement of CSF spaces occurs. Comparison with previous CT scans is wise when available. Although diffuse cerebral edema, by

Table 3				
Patterns of normal and pathological CSF spaces				
	Sulci	Fissures	Ventricles	Cisterns
Normal	Normal	Normal	Normal	Normal, including smile sign
Atrophy	Enlarged	Enlarged	Enlarged	Enlarged
Edema	Effaced	Effaced	Effaced	Effaced, including loss of smile sign
Hydrocephalus	Effaced	Effaced	Enlarged	Effaced, including loss of smile sign

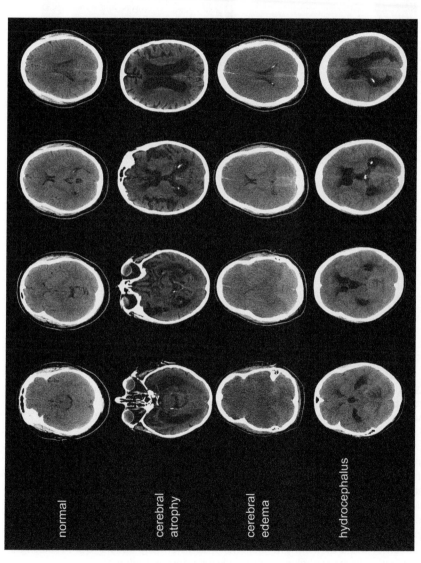

Fig. 22. An overview of the pattern of CSF spaces in normal and pathological conditions. For each row, left to right indicates caudal to rostral brain sections.

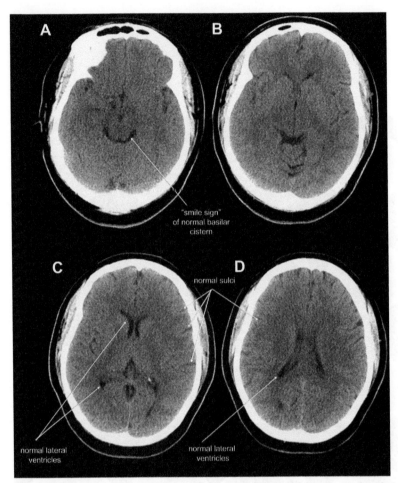

Fig. 23. A normal brain, without evidence of increased intracranial pressure. (*A–D*) Caudal to rostral brain sections. The ventricles and cisterns are open, neither slitlike nor enlarged. The sulci are visible but not prominent.

definition, should affect the entire brain, the rate of swelling may not be symmetrical. If expansion of structures results in compression of the third and fourth ventricles, cerebral aqueduct, or basilar cisterns, the route of egress of CSF from the remainder of the ventricular system may be cut off, and obstructive hydrocephalus may develop (discussed later). Thus, cerebral edema and hydrocephalus may coexist. In addition, subarachnoid hemorrhage (SAH) may coexist with cerebral edema. SAH can lead to obstruction of the arachnoid granulations, which normally absorb CSF, resulting in communicating hydrocephalus concurrently with cerebral edema.

CSF spaces alone suggest, but do not fully describe, the state of the brain. When diffuse cerebral edema occurs, in addition to effacement of CSF spaces, loss of gray-white matter differentiation may develop, as described earlier. Other traumatic injuries, including fractures and hemorrhage, may be present. However, diffuse cerebral edema may occur following trauma, in the absence of other injuries visible on CT. Several possible causes exist, including DAI, anoxic brain injury from airway

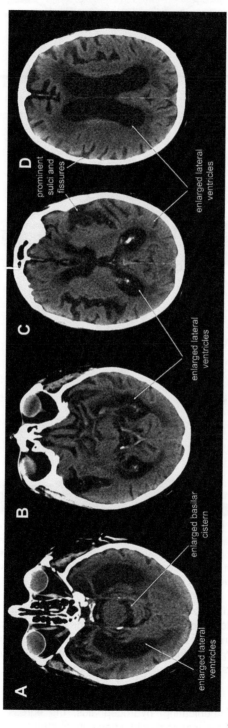

Fig. 24. Cerebral atrophy. In cerebral atrophy, all CSF spaces are enlarged, including ventricles, sulci and fissures, and cisterns. CSF fills available space as the brain volume decreases. (A–D) Caudal to rostral brain sections.

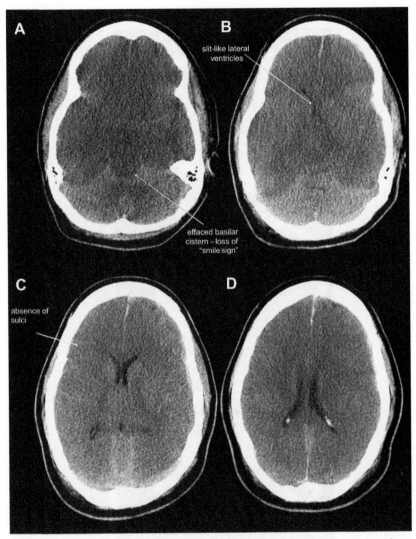

Fig. 25. Cerebral edema. In cerebral edema, the brain parenchyma increases in volume, at the expense of all CSF spaces. The cisterns and sulci are effaced, and ventricles become slit-like. No sulci are visible, and the smile sign of the normal basilar cistern (quadrigeminal plate cistern) is lost, a sign of uncal herniation. As discussed earlier, gray-white matter differentiation is lost. (*A–D*) Caudal to rostral brain sections.

occlusion, or prolonged hypotension from other traumatic injuries. Toxic exposures such as carbon monoxide and cyanide poisoning can occur with smoke or fire exposures, which may accompany trauma. These exposures can lead to secondary brain injury with diffuse edema. Often direct traumatic brain injury may be worsened by these secondary factors.

Hydrocephalus

In obstructive (noncommunicating) hydrocephalus, the egress of CSF from the ventricular system to the subarachnoid space is obstructed. In communicating hydrocephalus, the flow of CSF from the ventricles to the subarachnoid space is preserved, but absorption from the subarachnoid space is impaired. Both types of hydrocephalus may occur following trauma. Communicating hydrocephalus can result from subarachnoid hemorrhage if blood products in the subarachnoid spaced obstruct reabsorption of CSF by the arachnoid granulations.

The pattern of CSF spaces in hydrocephalus typically shows an increase in the size of the ventricles, whereas other CSF spaces are effaced because of the fixed total intracranial volume (**Fig. 26**; see also **Fig. 22**). Depending on the location of obstruction of CSF flow, upstream structures will be dilated and downstream structures will be decompressed. The normal route of CSF flow is shown in **Box 3**. The gross

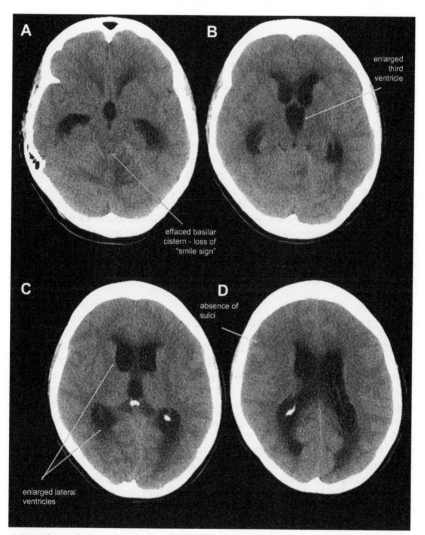

Fig. 26. Hydrocephalus. In hydrocephalus, the ventricles increase in size because of either increased CSF production, decreased reabsorption, or obstruction of flow. The sulci are obliterated and the cisterns become effaced, with the danger of ultimate uncal herniation. (*A–D*) Caudal to rostral brain sections.

Box 3
Normal route of CSF from production to clearance

Choroid plexus

Lateral ventricle

Interventricular foramen of Monro

Third ventricle

Cerebral aqueduct of Sylvius

Fourth ventricle

2 lateral foramina of Luschka and 1 medial foramen of Magendie

Subarachnoid space

Arachnoid granulations

Dural sinus

Venous drainage

---

appearance of the head CT with communicating hydrocephalus can resemble the face of a Halloween pumpkin. The large anterior horns of the lateral ventricles look like rounded eyes, whereas the normally slitlike third ventricle dilates to a rounded nose in the face. The smile sign of the quadrigeminal cistern may be effaced if downward herniation develops. However, the fourth ventricle (which lies just posterior to the quadrigeminal cistern) may become dilated, producing an O-shaped mouth in the face. The appearance has also been likened to a cartwheel, with 5 spokes (the 2 anterior and 2 posterior horns of the lateral ventricles, plus the fourth ventricle) radiating from an axle (the third ventricle). In noncommunicating hydrocephalus, the obstruction may lie above the level of the fourth ventricle, in which case the fourth ventricle will not appear dilated.

As described earlier, cerebral edema and other intracranial injuries may accompany hydrocephalus.

LIMITS OF CT AND THE ROLE OF MR IMAGING

Brain MRI is impractical in most acute emergency department trauma evaluations at this time, because of the time requirements and problems with monitoring patients with potentially unstable trauma in the MRI scanner. CT provides adequate information for most acute interventions and has similar sensitivity to MRI for hemorrhagic lesions. Studies of MRI suggest better detection of nonhemorrhagic lesions, with some caveats (discussed later). Future studies of MRI may reveal clinical benefits to patients, but this is not a foregone conclusion. The diagnostic power of MRI currently outstrips treatment options for traumatic brain injury, meaning that improved diagnosis may not be matched by improved neurological outcomes.

CT scan findings must always be placed in the context of the patient's clinical condition. Some patients seem surprisingly neurologically normal despite significant imaging abnormalities, and clinical decisions are based on multiple factors including the CT findings, the patient's condition, additional injuries and medical problems, and the anticipated course of the evolving injury. In other cases, a patient may seem neurologically devastated despite few abnormalities seen on CT. What accounts for this disparity between clinical condition and CT findings? How could 2 patients with similar CT findings have diametrically opposed neurological outcomes?

As described earlier, CT provides a view of brain anatomy based on tissue density differences. Some conditions do not substantially alter tissue densities, and CT is predictably poor in identifying these conditions, particularly early in their course. With time, secondary findings, such as diffuse cerebral edema or regional infarction, may develop and become visible with CT. Other factors, such as toxic exposures (alcohol, opiates, carbon monoxide, cyanide), may accompany trauma and may account for different neurological outcomes, in addition to traumatic brain injury itself.

DAI

DAI is a traumatic brain injury believed to occur primarily with high-velocity mechanisms of injury such as vehicle collisions and falls from great height. As the name implies, it is a diffuse brain injury to long axon tracts. Petechial brain hemorrhage and diffuse cerebral edema often accompany this injury, but the injury itself is invisible on CT, instead diagnosed by surrogate markers of hemorrhage and edema. The clinical presentation of severe DAI is a diffusely dysfunctional brain, with substantial degree of neurological impairment. Thus, a neurologically intact patient with a normal CT scan, or even with significant visible injury such as epidural hematoma, does not likely have DAI. MRI is believed to have significantly greater sensitivity and specificity for DAI than does noncontrast CT, although studies of this topic are limited, as described later. Currently, detection of this injury leads to little clinical action, because no specific therapy exists. The prognosis is poor, so confirmation with imaging may be important to long-term decisions about the patient's care.

Head CT may be normal in the presence of DAI, although large and methodologically rigorous studies do not exist. DAI is an injury diagnosed by pathological examination but, in studies of living patients, this is not feasible, so surrogates of DAI are often used. MRI produces exquisite images that may tempt clinicians to believe that their findings are always correct, but studies of MRI in other settings suggest that MRI can produce significant false-positive results. In a meta-analysis of MR mammography, 1 false-positive result occurred for every 2 true-positive studies.[38] Consequently, published studies of MRI accuracy for DAI without an independent diagnostic standard should be viewed skeptically. This article reviews some studies comparing the performance of CT with MRI for detection of DAI.

In 1988, Gentry and colleagues[39] performed a prospective study of CT and MRI in 40 patients with closed head injury and concluded that CT was only 19% sensitive for DAI, compared with 92% for T2-weighted MRI with axial and coronal reconstructions. However, this study used no independent standard for the diagnosis and thus suffers from incorporation bias (the use of a diagnostic study as its own gold standard, a well-described pitfall in research on diagnostic imaging).

IN 1994, Mittl and colleagues[40] examined the MRI findings in 20 patients with mild head injury (GCS 13–15) and normal head CT. Abnormalities compatible with DAI were seen in white matter in 30% (95% confidence interval 12%–54%). However, the small number of patients in this study, the absence of blinding, and the lack of an independent criterion standard limit the validity of this study. The investigators hypothesized that DAI seen on MRI may account for postconcussive symptoms in patients with normal CT.

In 2000, Paterakis and colleagues[41] reviewed MRI findings in 33 patients with normal CT but abnormal neurological examinations. Twenty-four patients had MRI findings compatible with DAI, again with no independent standard. In 2009, Skandsen and colleagues[42] compared 1-year outcomes in patients with moderate and severe head injury with and without DAI diagnosed by MRI. DAI was present in 72% of 106 patients but was associated with a negative outcome only when present within the brainstem. At this time, the clinical benefit of performing MRI is unclear, because no specific treatment of DAI exists.

SUMMARY

Noncontrast CT provides important diagnostic information for patients with traumatic brain injury. A systematic approach to image interpretation improves detection of pathological air, fractures, hemorrhagic lesions, brain parenchyma, and CSF spaces. Bone and brain windows should be reviewed to enhance injury detection. Findings of midline shift and mass effect should be noted as well as findings of increased intracranial pressure such as hydrocephalus and cerebral edema, because these may immediately influence management. Compared with CT, MRI may provide more sensitive detection of DAI but has no proven improvement in clinical outcomes.

REFERENCES

1. Raju TN. The Nobel chronicles. 1979: Allan MacLeod Cormack (b 1924); and Sir Godfrey Newbold Hounsfield (b 1919). Lancet 1999;354:1653.
2. New PF, Aronow S. Attenuation measurements of whole blood and blood fractions in computed tomography. Radiology 1976;121:635–40.
3. Smith WP Jr, Batnitzky S, Rengachary SS. Acute isodense subdural hematomas: a problem in anemic patients. AJR Am J Roentgenol 1981;136:543–6.
4. Subramanian SK, Roszler MH, Gaudy B, et al. Significance of computed tomography mixed density in traumatic extra-axial hemorrhage. Neurol Res 2002;24:125–8.
5. Choi HS, Choi BW, Choe KO, et al. Pitfalls, artifacts, and remedies in Multi-detector row CT coronary angiography1. Radiographics 2004;24:787–800.
6. Probst MA, Baraff LJ, Hoffman JR, et al. Can patients with brain herniation on cranial computed tomography have a normal neurologic exam? Acad Emerg Med 2009;16:145–50.
7. Bullock MR, Chesnut R, Ghajar J, et al. Surgical management of acute subdural hematomas. Neurosurgery 2006;58:S16–24 [discussion: Si–iv].
8. National Guideline Clearinghouse. Surgical management of acute epidural hematomas. Agency for Healthcare Research and Quality (AHRQ); 2006. Available at: http://www.guideline.gov/summary/summary.aspx?ss=15&doc_id=9439&nbr=5060#s25. Accessed May 5, 2010.
9. Bullock MR, Chesnut R, Ghajar J, et al. Surgical management of acute epidural hematomas. Neurosurgery 2006;58:S7–15 [discussion: Si–iv].
10. National Guideline Clearinghouse. Surgical management of acute subdural hematomas. Agency for Healthcare Research and Quality (AHRQ); 2006. Available at: http://www.guideline.gov/summary/summary.aspx?ss=15&doc_id=9440&nbr=5061. Accessed May 5, 2010.
11. Downer JJ, Pretorius PM. Symmetry in computed tomography of the brain: the pitfalls. Clin Radiol 2009;64:298–306.
12. Perron AD, Huff JS, Ullrich CG, et al. A multicenter study to improve emergency medicine residents' recognition of intracranial emergencies on computed tomography. Ann Emerg Med 1998;32:554–62.
13. Broder JS. Midnight radiology: head CT interpretation. 2006. Available at: www.emedhome.com. Accessed May 5, 2010.
14. Bhattacharyya N, Fried MP. The accuracy of computed tomography in the diagnosis of chronic rhinosinusitis. Laryngoscope 2003;113:125–9.

15. Bhattacharyya N, Jones DT, Hill M, et al. The diagnostic accuracy of computed tomography in pediatric chronic rhinosinusitis. Arch Otolaryngol Head Neck Surg 2004;130:1029–32.

16. Wittkopf ML, Beddow PA, Russell PT, et al. Revisiting the interpretation of positive sinus CT findings: a radiological and symptom-based review. Otolaryngol Head Neck Surg 2009;140:306–11.

17. Woodrow PK, Gajarawala J, Yaghoobian J, et al. CT detection of subarachnoid pneumocephalus secondary to mastoid fracture. J Comput Tomogr 1981;5: 199–201.

18. Sloan T. The incidence, volume, absorption, and timing of supratentorial pneumocephalus during posterior fossa neurosurgery conducted in the sitting position. J Neurosurg Anesthesiol 2010;22:59–66.

19. Syed ON, Weintraub D, DeLaPaz R, et al. Venous air emboli from intravenous catheterization: a report of iatrogenic intravascular pneumocephalus. J Clin Neurosci 2009;16:1361–2.

20. Jagoda AS, Bazarian JJ, Bruns JJ Jr, et al. Clinical policy: neuroimaging and decisionmaking in adult mild traumatic brain injury in the acute setting. Ann Emerg Med 2008;52:714–48.

21. American College of Radiology. ACR Appropriateness Criteria: head trauma. 2008. Available at: http://www.acr.org/SecondaryMainMenuCategories/quality_safety/app_criteria/pdf/ExpertPanelonNeurologicImaging/HeadTraumaDoc5.aspx. Accessed May 3, 2008.

22. Skull fracture: treatment. 2009. Available at: http://emedicine.medscape.com/article/248108-treatment. Accessed May 5, 2010.

23. Demetriades D, Charalambides D, Lakhoo M, et al. Role of prophylactic antibiotics in open and basilar fractures of the skull: a randomized study. Injury 1992;23:377–80.

24. Ratilal B, Costa J, Sampaio C. Antibiotic prophylaxis for preventing meningitis in patients with basilar skull fractures. Cochrane Database Syst Rev 2006;1: CD004884.

25. Erlichman DB, Blumfield E, Rajpathak S, et al. Association between linear skull fractures and intracranial hemorrhage in children with minor head trauma. Pediatr Radiol 2010;40:1375–9.

26. Boesiger BM, Shiber JR. Subarachnoid hemorrhage diagnosis by computed tomography and lumbar puncture: are fifth generation CT scanners better at identifying subarachnoid hemorrhage? J Emerg Med 2005;29:23–7.

27. Byyny RL, Mower WR, Shum N, et al. Sensitivity of noncontrast cranial computed tomography for the Emergency Department diagnosis of subarachnoid hemorrhage. Ann Emerg Med 2008;51:697–703.

28. Noguchi K, Seto H, Kamisaki Y, et al. Comparison of fluid-attenuated inversion-recovery MR imaging with CT in a simulated model of acute subarachnoid hemorrhage. AJNR Am J Neuroradiol 2000;21:923–7.

29. Callaway CW. Why does the sensitivity of computed tomographic scan for detecting subarachnoid blood never improve? Ann Emerg Med 2008;51:705–6.

30. Gentleman D, Nath F, Macpherson P. Diagnosis and management of delayed traumatic intracerebral haematomas. Br J Neurosurg 1989;3:367–72.

31. Huisman TA, Tschirch FT. Epidural hematoma in children: do cranial sutures act as a barrier? J Neuroradiol 2009;36:93–7.

32. Al-Nakshabandi NA. The swirl sign. Radiology 2001;218:433.

33. Zimmerman RA, Bilaniuk LT. Computed tomographic staging of traumatic epidural bleeding. Radiology 1982;144:809–12.

34. Greenberg J, Cohen WA, Cooper PR. The "hyperacute" extraaxial intracranial hematoma: computed tomographic findings and clinical significance. Neurosurgery 1985;17:48–56.
35. Pruthi N, Balasubramaniam A, Chandramouli BA, et al. Mixed-density extradural hematomas on computed tomography-prognostic significance. Surg Neurol 2009;71:202–6.
36. Holodny AI, Visvikis GA, Schlenk RP, et al. Bilateral subdural hematomas exactly isodense to the subjacent gray matter. J Emerg Med 2001;20:413–4.
37. Parizel PM, Ozsarlak, Van Goethem JW, et al. Imaging findings in diffuse axonal injury after closed head trauma. Eur Radiol 1998;8:960–5.
38. Houssami N, Ciatto S, Macaskill P, et al. Accuracy and surgical impact of magnetic resonance imaging in breast cancer staging: systematic review and meta-analysis In detection of multifocal and multicentric cancer. J Clin Oncol 2008;26:3248–58.
39. Gentry LR, Godersky JC, Thompson B, et al. Prospective comparative study of intermediate-field MR and CT in the evaluation of closed head trauma. AJR Am J Roentgenol 1988;150:673–82.
40. Mittl RL, Grossman RI, Hiehle JF, et al. Prevalence of MR evidence of diffuse axonal injury in patients with mild head injury and normal head CT findings. AJNR Am J Neuroradiol 1994;15:1583–9.
41. Paterakis K, Karantanas AH, Komnos A, et al. Outcome of patients with diffuse axonal injury: the significance and prognostic value of MRI in the acute phase. J Trauma 2000;49:1071–5.
42. Skandsen T, Kvistad KA, Solheim O, et al. Prevalence and impact of diffuse axonal injury in patients with moderate and severe head injury: a cohort study of early magnetic resonance imaging findings and 1-year outcome. J Neurosurg 2010;113:556–63.

Neuropsychological Assessment in Traumatic Brain Injury

Kenneth Podell, PhD[a,b,]*, Katherine Gifford, PsyD[a],
Dmitri Bougakov, PhD[c], Elkhonon Goldberg, PhD[d]

KEYWORDS

- Traumatic brain injury • Executive control
- Neuropsychological testing

Neuropsychology is a hybrid science of brain-behavior relationships, drawing expertise from psychology, psychiatry, and neurology. Clinical neuropsychology uses "psychological, neurological, behavioral, and physiological techniques and tests to evaluate the patients' neurocognitive, behavioral, and emotional strengths and weaknesses and their relationship to normal and abnormal central nervous system functioning.[1]" By incorporating the history, patient's presentation, medical findings, and neuropsychological test scores, the neuropsychologist's aim is to link cognition, behavior, and emotion to brain anatomy and function.[2] The goal of a clinical neuropsychological evaluation is multifactorial and can assist the patient or referring health care provider to better understand differential diagnosis, cognitive/behavioral strengths and weaknesses as they relate to the disease and syndrome or injury of interest, as well as to develop interventional strategies and recommendations.

Clinical neuropsychology is particularly important in measuring cognitive and emotional dysfunction following neurological insult or disruption, such as traumatic brain injury (TBI). To do this, neuropsychologists employ techniques or tests (usually paper-and-pencil and computerized tests) that allow for measuring behavior. Neuropsychological assessment represents a crucial component of neuropsychology, as it remains one of the most effective means for determining the current level of cognitive functioning in an individual.[3] Clinical neuropsychology is an intricate component in

[a] Division of Neuropsychology, Henry Ford Health System, One Ford Place–1E, Detroit, MI 48322, USA
[b] Department of Psychiatry, Wayne State University, Detroit, MI, USA
[c] City University of New York, NY, USA
[d] Department of Neurology, New York University School of Medicine, 550 First Avenue, New York, NY 10016, USA
* Corresponding author. Division of Neuropsychology, Henry Ford Health System, One Ford Place–1E, Detroit, MI 48322.
E-mail address: KPODELL1@HFHS.org

Psychiatr Clin N Am 33 (2010) 855–876
doi:10.1016/j.psc.2010.08.003
0193-953X/10/$ – see front matter © 2010 Elsevier Inc. All rights reserved.

psych.theclinics.com

diagnosing, developing treatment programs, and monitoring recovery of TBI. This article introduces the field of neuropsychology and outlines the role, utility, and process of neuropsychological assessment within the TBI population. Expected neuropsychological deficits associated with both level of TBI severity and time following the injury are explored. Lastly, there is a discussion of other factors associated with a TBI that can affect neuropsychological performance.

ROLE OF NEUROPSYCHOLOGY IN TBI

TBI is not only the most common brain injury/disease but also one of the more heterogeneous. TBI can result in graded neurological, physical, emotional, and neuropsychological changes and deficits that are dependent on the injury severity; however, it should be emphasized that the Glasgow Coma Scale (GCS) score itself does not necessarily predict the degree of injury or consequent dysfunction. Preexisting psychological and psychosocial factors, as well as several post-incident factors and support systems, may contribute to the TBI recovery process. Neuropsychology contributes uniquely through the assessment process by providing a holistic approach, by measuring cognitive and emotional deficits, and by identifying the etiology of these deficits (eg, TBI vs other confounding variables associated with a traumatic event). Neuropsychologists consider a wide range of factors beyond the manifestations of the TBI; specifically, premorbid functioning is considered with respect to post-injury neuropsychological functioning, as are psychosocial factors such as emotional well-being and social support. Using this holistic approach, neuropsychology is better able to direct treatment and inform about prognosis. Overall, neuropsychological assessment serves a multitude of purposes in TBI: diagnostic, treatment planning, evaluating treatment progression, forensic assessment, and research. A recent study found that TBI severity alone accounted for only a small percentage (5%) of the variance in neuropsychological test performance, particularly for mild TBI.[4] In addition, when considering functional status, cognitive abilities account for 21% to 30% of the variance.[5] These results indicate the importance for the neuropsychologist to consider the presence of other factors that may play a role in the deficits commonly seen in individuals with TBI.

Age

Age is an important factor, as younger and older brains are more vulnerable to the effects of TBI. Young children and older adults are at greater risk of experiencing long-term cognitive deficits than older children and younger adults.[6-8]

Multiple TBIs

A history of prior TBI increases the likelihood of cognitive deficits from subsequent events.[9,10] The sports concussion literature has shown that individuals with a prior history of concussions (usually 3 or more) are more likely to evidence concussion-related symptoms and neuropsychological deficits on subsequent events and even long term.[11,12]

Depression

Although on review of the literature approximately 14% to 61% of individuals with TBI have been reported to experience depressed mood during their first year after injury,[5,13,14] most of the studies are flawed and encumbered by bias, thus more research is needed. Also, a clear distinction needs to be made between depressed mood in the setting of TBI versus meeting full Axis I criteria for major depression: Determining if the depressed mood is situational, secondary to a structural lesion, or secondary to a primary mood disorder or to a medical condition is often difficult and requires a detailed assessment. Gasquoine[15] reported increased emotional distress that predicted the presence of persistent symptomatology following TBI. However, patients with depression, but without TBI, have similar symptom reporting and cognitive deficits to TBI patients.[16,17] Cognitively, individuals with depression can demonstrate neuropsychological impairment within the areas of attention, executive functioning, memory, and psychomotor speed; exactly the same as found for TBI. Thus, patients who have recovered from a mild TBI but are depressed may have a similar symptom profile and cognitive deficits to patients with cognitive deficits from TBI alone, continuing however to attribute them to TBI. Moreover, report of pain, sleep disturbance, and side effects of medication can all worsen depressive symptoms and neuropsychological deficits after TBI.

Posttraumatic Stress Disorder

There is much overlap in the symptoms and cognitive deficits of posttraumatic stress disorder (PTSD) and TBI. Both PTSD and TBI are associated with neuropsychological deficits of attention, particularly working memory.[18] Memory disorders associated with PTSD are caused by deficits in attention, which interfere with the encoding and consolidation of new information[19] as similarly found in TBI. Given the degree of overlap in symptomatology, the clinical neuropsychologist must include objective measures and data to ensure accurate diagnoses and prevent over- and misdiagnoses of either condition.[20]

Psychiatric History

Understanding premorbid personality factors and underlying psychopathology is important in predicting outcome and planning treatment. Specifically, an individual's ability to adjust and cope with the changes associated with a TBI is linked to premorbid personality factors.[7] There is some evidence to suggest less importance of a history of psychiatric disturbance in the outcome from TBI. Mooney and Speed[21] suggested no relationship between prior psychiatric history and outcome from mild TBI. Similarly, they indicated that those with a previous history of psychiatric disturbance were not more likely to have psychiatric disturbance following a TBI.

Substance Abuse

Alcohol and substance abuse are common premorbid factors in individuals who suffer from TBI. Cognitive deficits associated with substance abuse are similar to those found in TBI. For example, alcohol abuse can disrupt executive functioning, with additional problems with learning and perceptual-motor dysfunction.[22] Similarly, chronic opiate abuse has been linked to deficits in executive functioning and working memory.[23] Of note, individuals with a mild TBI do not differ on neuropsychological performance as compared with individuals with a history of substance abuse.[24] Thus, it can be difficult to differentiate the cause of the post-TBI cognitive deficits in those with a preexisting history of substance abuse.

Effort

Test invalidity in neuropsychological assessment can be seen in 2 ways: (1) individuals not motivated to perform and thus not "trying hard" and (2) individuals attempting to exaggerate impairment by answering incorrectly or feigning deficits. One could argue in the latter case that these individuals are in fact being highly effortful, as it would seem to take more effort to think of the right answer but then change it to give the incorrect answer. Poor effort can be caused by factors other than TBI (premorbid or post-incident factors) such as secondary gain. However, individuals with true neurological insult can demonstrate poor effort due to legitimate factors. Regardless of the rationale for poor effort, measuring effort is essential in TBI, as approximately 40% of people with mild TBI have exaggerated symptoms during assessment.[25] Effort is a clear mediator of neuropsychological performance, accounting for a greater proportion of the variance on neuropsychological performance than the severity of TBI itself.[4,26] Neuropsychological performance deemed invalid due to poor effort should not be immediately considered a product of feigning or malingering.[27]

Pain

One large confounding factor of TBI is pain, especially considering TBI most often occurs in conjunction with physical injuries, particularly to the back and neck, with headache being the most commonly reported symptom.[20] Chronic pain, including headaches, is associated with deficits in neuropsychological performance within the domains of working memory/attention and psychomotor speed.[29,30]

Litigation Status

Litigation status is an important, albeit controversial, factor in recovery from TBI.[7,31] Litigation status involves individuals who are seeking financial compensation for residual injuries following a TBI. This type of post-incident factor[32] can create a clinical syndrome in someone without any residual deficits, or distort a true clinical picture such that deficits and symptoms that normally would recover continue to be reported over time.[33,34] Litigation is a prominent and consistent factor accounting for poor outcome and prolonged recovery from mild TBI.[25,35–37] Individuals seeking financial compensation are 4 times more likely to give poor effort on neuropsychological testing,[27] with other studies reporting about a 40% base rate of poor effort/test invalidity in personal injury cases.[38–40] Others have found that those in litigation presented with greater subjective complaints and did worse on neuropsychological performance than nonlitigating mild TBI individuals matched for injury severity.[8,41] Moreover, mild TBI patients seeking compensation take more medications and report twice the symptoms as matched nonlitigating mild TBI patients.[42] Thus, litigation status may mediate the profile of neuropsychological performance and symptoms, and the presence of active litigation should be carefully considered when determining the etiology of cognitive impairment seen following TBI. Though unclear, there is likely an admixture of iatrogenic factors and intentionality accounting for these differences.

PROCESS OF NEUROPSYCHOLOGICAL ASSESSMENT

The neuropsychological evaluation in the TBI patient requires a comprehensive approach to assess most cognitive domains, psychiatric symptoms, psychological factors, and psychosocial variables and functioning. The evaluation must assess both acute and chronic deficits to best predict functional outcome and ability.[7] The evaluation is key in working through the differential diagnosis of post-TBI presentation and provides the basis for constructing the therapeutic strategy.[43] Neuropsychological performance has been linked with functional status 6 months after injury, and with ability to return to work and employment outcomes.[5,44,45]

The specific battery of tests is often determined by the severity of the injury, patient's age, and the duration of time after injury. For example, individuals with severe TBI and persistent functional deficits will often receive a shorter battery of tests that is not as difficult to complete in order to prevent fatigue and a flooring effect. Conversely, an individual with mild TBI will typically receive a more comprehensive battery of neuropsychological tests with a wider range of complexity and difficulty so as to detect subtle deficits.[7] The utility of neuropsychological testing is generally more helpful with mild to moderate TBI, as these individuals generally improve, often back to baseline functioning.

Neuropsychological assessment uses tests that allow for a comparison of the brain-injured individual to healthy subjects matched along various demographic variables, for example, age, education, and gender, or to known clinical groups, for example, with TBI or other conditions.[3] The neuropsychological evaluation typically consists of a comprehensive and detailed clinical interview with the patient, review of medical records, gathering of collateral information (interview(s) with family members), test selection, test administration, scoring and interpretation of test results, recommendations, and feedback to the patient, all of which are clearly described in a formal report.

In moderate and severe TBI, the earliest neuropsychological assessment often occurs during inpatient hospitalization. The Galveston Orientation and Amnesia Test (GOAT)[46] is a repeatable test of confusion and amnesia used to determine when a patient's posttraumatic amnesia (PTA) has resolved. The GOAT score determines when a patient is capable of undergoing more formal neuropsychological assessment. The GOAT provides a standardized and quantitative method for assessing the length of PTA, which is important because length of PTA can be crucial in helping to predict outcome from TBI. Specifically, in severe TBI the length of PTA as measured by the GOAT was correlated with outcome at 6 months after injury.[46,47] Exactly when to perform more extensive inpatient or outpatient neuropsychological testing is determined by multiple factors including TBI severity, reason for the assessment, pain, side effects of medication, emotional factors, and so forth.

Fixed Versus Flexible Battery

Once a TBI patient is ready for more formal and extensive neuropsychological testing, the clinical neuropsychologist can use a "fixed" or a more "flexible" battery of neuropsychological testing (**Box 1**). In a fixed battery approach, the neuropsychologist administers the same test instruments to every patient in a standard manner regardless of the patient's presenting illness, referral question, or background.[48] The most popular neuropsychological battery is The Halstead-Reitan Neuropsychological Battery (HRNB).[7,49] Advantages of the fixed battery approach to neuropsychological assessment include: (1) it provides a comprehensive assessment of multiple cognitive domains; and (2) it uses a standardized format that allows the test data to be incorporated into databases for clinical and scientific analysis. Disadvantages of the fixed battery approach include (1) time and labor intensiveness; and (2) a lack of flexibility in different clinical situations; specifically, multiple, nonequivalent data sets exist and specific normative data with TBI patients should be used with caution.[48,50–52]

In using a flexible approach to neuropsychological testing, individual tests are chosen based on the patient's presenting illness or referral question.[7,53,54] Primary advantages of the flexible approach to neuropsychological evaluation include: (1) a potentially shorter administration time; (2) economical favorability; and (3) adaptability to differing patient situations and needs. Some [53,55] argue that the flexible approach permits better specification of the deficits within a given cognitive domain as well as their underlying neural systems rather than simply documenting the presence or absence of brain damage. Others use the flexible approach because it permits easy evaluation of qualitative features such as the patient's use of problem-solving strategies.[56] Finally, test modification inherent in the flexible approach makes it adaptable to a wide variety of clinical situations,[48] which is useful given the heterogeneity of TBI. Disadvantages of the flexible approach include: (1) the need for greater clinical

---

Box 1
Example of a fixed battery

Halstead-Reitan Battery

    Tactual performance test

        Total time

        Localization

        Memory

    Finger oscillation test (dominant hand)

    Category test

    Seashore rhythm test

    Speech sounds perception test

    Aphasia screening test

    Sensory-perceptual examination

    Strength of grip test

    Tactile form recognition test

Data from Heaton RK, Grant I, Matthews CG. Comprehensive norms for an expanded Halstead-Reitan battery. Odessa (FL): Psychological Assessment Resources; 1991.

---

experience; (2) a lack of standardized administration rules for some tests; (3) a potential lack of comprehensiveness; and (4) limitations in establishing systematic databases.[48,57] An understanding of developmental normal aging, age-related cognitive decline, neuropsychological principles, neuropathological conditions, and other issues pertinent to differential diagnosis are particularly important when using the flexible neuropsychological assessment approach with TBI. However, this individualized approach to neuropsychological assessment remains popular with many neuropsychologists because of its adaptability, flexibility, clinical usefulness of qualitative information, efficiency with severely impaired patients, and applicability with patients who are vulnerable to fatigue, distress, or sensory limitations.[48,58]

Estimates of Pre-Injury Abilities

An important "first step" in the neuropsychological assessment of TBI involves estimating the individual's pre-injury level of ability and cognitive functioning using a combination of demographic variables and actual test performances. This approach is useful in determining whether a decline has occurred in the current test performance. Various demographic variables influence neuropsychological test performance. For example, gender can play a role in neuropsychological performance, with females often performing better on verbal tasks and males better on spatial tasks.[7] However, education is the premorbid factor with the most powerful effect on neuropsychological performance.[7,59] The positive relationship is greatest for verbal-based skills, but is often found for any type of neuropsychological performance. Educational attainment and occupational functioning obviously are strong predictors of pre-injury functioning. Grade attainment may not be the most accurate indicator, as a wide range of ability exists within each grade level. Also, patients can overestimate their educational attainment or grade point average (GPA).[60] To that end, obtaining school records, including standardized scores, GPA, and so forth can help more accurately predict pre-injury level of functioning. Moreover, GPA correlated with post-TBI neuropsychological test performance in cases of mild TBI.[61] Employment type and level can also help predict pre-injury functional levels. Apart from records and self-report, there are direct testing methods used to help estimate pre-injury ability level. One of the more common techniques is single word reading recognition. The reading recognition subtest from The Wide Range Achievement Test (now in fourth edition) and The North American Adult Reading Test,[62] for example, are commonly employed to this end.[7]

NEUROPSYCHOLOGICAL DOMAINS

The formal neuropsychological assessment in TBI assesses a wide variety of areas including estimates of pre-injury abilities, test engagement, formal neuropsychological domains, psychiatric status, and emotional functioning (**Box 2**).

Language and Speech

Alterations in language and speech following TBI often vary depending on severity of TBI and location of focal lesions. Focal dominant hemisphere lesions (left in normally lateralized individuals) may require formal aphasia assessment. However, typically in TBI, word finding problems (anomia) may be more common. Verbal fluency is commonly evaluated in TBI. Verbal fluency measures can assess for fluency rate and semantic accessing (word finding) as well as executive control components (see later discussion).

Visuospatial/Construction

A wide variety of skills fall under visuospatial and construction. Typically, these tasks require an understanding of spatial relationships between component parts, assuming basic perceptual abilities are intact. However, the output mode on these tasks is important. Motor and executive components are often intermixed with spatial aspects in constructional tasks. Nonmotoric spatial tasks, on the other hand, tend not to have a strong executive component per se. For example, The Rey-Osterrieth Complex Figure Test[7] involves copying a complex design. This test has both a strong visuospatial and executive control component, whereas a task such as Benton's Test of Spatial Orientation,[63] whereby the subject has to match a pair of corresponding lines from a template of 11 lines arranged in a 180° arc to 2 stimuli lines of various angles, does not have as strong an executive control component.

Attention/Concentration

Individuals with TBI are vulnerable to deficits in attention and concentration, particularly in the acute stage of the injury. Attention and concentration consist of a rubric of neuropsychological functions that tend to build on each other. For example, general arousal is the most basic aspect, followed by general orientation. A detailed assessment of attention is important because all other neuropsychological abilities build on it; if a patient cannot sustain his or her attention, impaired performance on a memory test may actually represent an attentional deficit. The assessment of attention often starts with attentional span, that is, how much information the person can take in at once. Digit or spatial spans from The Wechsler Scales[64,65] are commonly used for this. Assessing for level of distractibility via sustained attention or vigilance is important, and is accomplished with computerized continuous performance tests or speeded cancellation paradigms. Speed of information processing also falls under attentional processes, and tasks that measure throughput (speed and accuracy of response) are particularly sensitive to this. Examples of this are Digit Symbol from the Wechsler

---

Box 2
Cognitive domains and representative neuropsychological tests[a]

Attention.

    Digit span (Wechsler Adult Intelligence Scale——III & Wechsler Memory Scale—— III).

    Letter-number sequencing (Wechsler Adult Intelligence Scale——III & Wechsler Memory Scale—— III).

    Visual memory span (spatial span, Wechsler Memory Scale—III-WMS-III).

    Cancellation tests (number, letter, or figure).

    Continuous Performance Test.

    Stroop Test.

    Trail Making Test.

Memory (Immediate and Delayed Recall and Recognition).

    Wechsler Memory Scale—IIIWMS-III (Psychological Corporation).

    California Verbal Learning Test——II.

    Rey-Osterrieth Complex Figure Test.

    Rey Auditory-Verbal Learning Test.

Executive Functions.

    Category Test.

    Wisconsin Card Sorting Test.

    Trail Making Test.

    Stroop Test.

    Executive Control Battery.

    Delis-Kaplan Executive Functions System.

Language.

    Boston Diagnostic Aphasia Examination.

    Multilingual Aphasia Examination.

    Reitan-Indiana Aphasia Screening Test.

    Word fluency (semantic/categorical and phonemic/letter).

Visuospatial and Visuomotor Processes.

    Facial recognition test.

    Judgment of line orientation.

    Visual form discrimination test.

    Benton Visual Retention Test.

    Rey-Osterrieth Complex Figure (copy).

Motor Processes.

    Finger oscillation test.

    Grooved pegboard test.

    Purdue Pegboard Test.

    Strength of grip test

Affect and Personality.

Minnesota Multiphasic Personality Assessment.

Beck Inventories (Depression and Anxiety).

Personality Assessment Inventory.

Symptom checklist—90 questions.

Effort (Imbedded and Free-standing)

Word memory test.

Tests of memory malingering.

Reliable digit and spatial span.

Dot counting test.

[a] The measures listed are considered representative of the domain and are not intended to be definitive measures.

Adult Intelligence Scale, and speeded cancellation tests. Measures of divided attention (ability to perform 2 tasks at once) can be assessed; this would include tasks such as The Auditory Consonant Trigram Test (or Brown-Peterson paradigm) and The Paced Auditory Serial Addition Test. Lastly, working memory, or the ability to hold information "on-line" and manipulate it, is typical in the neuropsychological assessment of TBI. Typical examples are Digit or Spatial Span Backwards and Letter/Number Sequencing (from the Wechsler Scales).

Memory

Memory problems are the most common complaint after TBI. Memory, specifically anterograde memory, is a multifaceted ability to learn, retain, recall, and recognize new information. The typical paradigms used in neuropsychological assessment ask the patient to learn new information and to recall it immediately after presentation, later typically 20 to 30 minutes after presentation (delayed recall), and followed by a delayed recognition component. Multiple modalities and formats are used to assess anterograde memory. First, material can be verbal (often presented auditorially) or spatial (nonmeaningful visual material). For verbal material short paragraphs, word pairs, and word lists are typically employed. Some of the memory tasks only allow for single presentation, whereas others repeat the material over multiple presentations to assess learning. Some tasks incorporate distractor material to assess for interference effects. After a specific period of time, short- and long-delay recall are used to assess for level of memory storage or retention. Lastly, recognition, using a yes/no recognition or multiple-choice paradigms, are used to assess recognition. Incorporating all of these components allows the neuropsychologist to assess different aspects of memory and the integrity of the neuroanatomical structures involved in memory.

Executive Control

Executive control is the most complex and elusive neuropsychological domain,[7,66] encompassing a multitude of abilities that involve mental planning, organization, adaptation to novelty, shifting of cognitive set, reasoning, and error monitoring, to name a few. One does not have to injure directly the prefrontal regions—the neuroanatomical area responsible for executive control skills—to induce executive control deficits.[66] Numerous, nonfocal injuries or disease states, including TBI, can produce executive deficits.[7,66] Ubiquitous across all neuropsychological domains, executive control functions are an integral component of any formal neuropsychological assessment, which is why the authors believe that assessment of executive dysfunction requires special attention and thus dedicate an entire section to its detailed discussion later in this article.

Although there are numerous tests specifically designed to assess executive function, it is detectable on numerous "nonexecutive" measures such as memory.[67] Executive control components commonly assessed in TBI include planning, deductive reasoning and problem solving, set shifting, generativity and fluency, and error monitoring. Also, behavioral and personality changes associated with injury to the orbitfrontal region of the brain can occur following TBI. Various self-report and collateral questionnaires exist to help the clinician assess these changes (Frontal System Behavior Scale and Behavior Rating Inventory of Executive Functions).

Sensory and Motor

Sensory and motor skills are considered part of a comprehensive neuropsychological assessment. These skills typically are not affected in mild TBI (unless spinal injury is involved) and are directly related to injury to primary motor and sensory regions and cerebellum, but can be related to slower processing speed in more severe cases of TBI. Skills such as motor speed, dexterity, and strength are used to assess motor integrity, whereas tactile, visual, and auditory sensation, integration, and inattention are assessed for the sensory abilities.

Affect and Personality

The assessment of personality variables, mood, affect, and self-report symptoms are integral in understanding the effects of TBI. Lengthy self-report questionnaires (eg, The Minnesota Multiphasic Personality Inventory) are used to detect and tease apart the emotional, psychological, and psychiatric components often found in TBI. These questionnaires are helpful in assessing the individual's self-report in terms of mood, affect, pain, cognitive complaints, psychological variables and personality components, and reaction to his or her injury.

EXECUTIVE FUNCTIONS IN TBI

The executive functions and its substrate the frontal lobes are affected in a variety of clinical conditions and are vulnerable in TBI,[68,69] either in the presence of a focal lesion or not. Frontal lobe dysfunctions in TBI can be secondary to direct frontal injury or injury disrupting the reticular-frontal connection. In addition to the frontal lobes, other neuroanatomic structures can have a role in the executive control: These structures include the anterior cingulate cortex, basal ganglia, possibly the dorsomedial thalamic nucleus, cerebellum, and ventral mesencephalon. Frontal lobe syndromes accompanied by pronounced hypofrontality[70] can be seen even in the cases of TBI even in the absence of evidence of structural damage to the frontal lobes on neuroimaging, thus emphasizing the important role of neuropsychological testing in the evaluation of these patients.

The concept of executive control constitutes a construct that is based on the cognitive symptoms of the frontal lobe disorder caused by many different underlying conditions, thus no single measure of executive functions is adequate. Therefore, in the assessment of a patient who has suffered a TBI it is necessary to administer several complementary tests of executive function. Utilization of these measures provides an adequate, though relatively straightforward, mechanism in assessing executive systems dysfunction. However, additional innovative procedures have been introduced recently such as the Cognitive Bias Task (CBT) and the Iowa Gambling Test (IGT). These tests can help the clinician better assess the patient's decision-making capacity and therefore determine ability to be employed and best employable option for the patient.

The Nature of Executive Functions

To better understand the frontal lobe, its function and dysfunction, and the role of working memory, one has to be aware of the work of Alexander Luria, Joaquin Fuster, and Patricia Goldman-Rakic. It was Luria[71] who in 1966 proposed the existence of a system in charge of intentionality, the formulation of goals, the plans of action subordinate to the goals, the identification of goal-appropriate cognitive routines, the sequential access to these routines, the temporally ordered transition from one routine to another, and the editorial evaluation of the outcome of our actions. He linked 2 broad types of cognitive operations to the executive control system: (1) the organism's ability to guide its behavior by internal representations[72]; (2) mental flexibility, the capacity to respond rapidly to unanticipated environmental contingencies, an ability to shift cognitive set.[73]

Joaquin Fuster[74] enlarged on Lurian definition by suggesting that the so-called executive systems can be considered functionally "homogeneous" in the sense that they are in charge of actions, both external and internal, for example, logical reasoning. The concept of executive function appears to be a multifactorial and not a unitary construct. It includes the following components: goal setting, cognitive tool selection, cognitive switching and mental flexibility, evaluating outcome, and adapting the current plan of execution appropriately. In patients who undergo a TBI, these functions can be compromised with subsequent neurobehavioral impairment and/or a different degree of functional impairment. To optimize patient functions, possible neurobehavioral sequelae and/or physical/neurological impairment needs to be understood and framed in the setting of the injury itself: the patient's baseline cognitive abilities, defense mechanisms, and presence or lack of social support must be taken into consideration; this would allow for early intervention when needed, and the establishment of behavioral strategies and psychotherapeutic and/or pharmacological interventions to help recovery.

Neuropsychological Measures of Executive Functions

A variety of neuropsychological tests are used in the assessment of frontal lobe function and dysfunction; among them a family of Tower tests, the Wisconsin Card Sorting Test (WCST), Category Test, and a family of Stroop tests[7] stand out.

Tower tests are a family of somewhat similar tests, among which the towers of London,[75] Hanoi, and Toronto[7] are most frequently used. The Tower tests measure the ability to plan ahead. The subjects are required to build a tower or a pyramid according to a prespecified arrangement of pieces.

The Wisconsin Card Sorting and Category Test

The WCST, developed by Grant and Berg,[76] assesses mental flexibility, the ability to use feedback to shift cognitive sets, and goal-directed behavior.[7] The WCST challenges the ability to develop and maintain an appropriate problem-solving strategy in the face of changing conditions in order to achieve a goal. Respondents are required to sort the cards according to different principles during the test administration. The Category Test was first described by Halstead and Settlage[77] and in its original form is a part of the HRNB. It also challenges problem-solving ability. Respondents are required to determine an underlying principle that can be used to categorize geometric figures based on feedback.

Stroop and flanker tests

The family of Stroop[78,79] and Eriksen flanker tests[80,81] measures freedom from distractibility, selective attention, ability to resolve response conflict, and response inhibition. The Stroop tests are based on the phenomenon that it takes longer to name colors than to read words and even longer to name the color of the ink in which a color name is printed when they are different.[78,82] Patients with frontal lesions have been shown to perform worse on Stroop test than those with posterior lesions.[83] A typical version of a Stroop test consists of 3 trials: word reading, color naming, and an interference trial in which the first two are a baseline measure and the third is a critical measure, whereby respondents are required to name the color of the ink in which a color name is printed when they are different.

A typical version of the Eriksen flanker test is visual task whereby the participant is instructed to respond to a centered and directed item flanked by distracting symbols such as arrows or letters. The symbols are called "congruent" if they all point in the same direction, the subject will have a short reaction time, and performance is more exact. Flanking arrows that point to a different direction are therefore incongruent and correspond to a slower reaction time and less accurate performance. Performance on these tasks has been linked to the function of the anterior cingulated cortex and has been shown to be impaired even in mild TBI.[84]

"Hot" versus "cool" executive functions

More recently a distinction has been made between the "cool" and the "hot" affective aspects of executive functions.[85,86] The "cool" (without reward/penalty) cognitive aspects of executive functions, more associated with dorsolateral regions of prefrontal cortex, could be measured, for example, by WCST and Tower tests. The "hot" affective (with reward/penalty) aspects, more associated with ventral and medial regions, could be measured, for example, by the IGT[87] and its variants.[88] It is plausible that this additional line of inquiry in the nature of executive function will contribute to development of new and original neuropsychological measures of frontal lobe dysfunction.

Executive Control Batteries

Among several batteries of executive control evaluation that exist, the Delis-Kaplan Executive Function System (D-KEFS)[89] and the Executive Control Battery (ECB)[90] are worth mentioning in detail.

The ECB[90] is a neuropsychological battery aimed to document the presence and the extent of certain qualitative features of "executive dysfunction." The battery is based on approaches and procedures developed and used by Alexander Luria and Elkhonon Goldberg; it is useful in eliciting pathognomic signs. The ECB is unique in the way that it combines qualitative and quantitative measurements by preserving traditional Lurian qualitative type of error analysis while adding quantitative analysis. The ECB was designed to elicit the various qualitative manifestations of the executive dysfunction (ie, perseverations, echopraxia, field-dependent behavior, inertia, stereotypies, and so forth) through standard, quantitative procedures. Various qualitative types of deficits are identified and their magnitude is quantified. The battery therefore combines the advantages of qualitative and quantitative psychometric approaches, enabling one to elicit and score errors in a standardized and quantitative fashion. The ECB consists of 4 subtests each known to be capable of eliciting the particular features of executive dysfunction. These subtests are the graphical sequence test, the competing programs test, the manual postures test, and the graphic sequences test. In preliminary data, Podell and Lovell[91] showed that mirroring errors on the manual postures subtest were at least as accurate in discriminating healthy controls from the TBI group as WCST perseverative responses. In addition, Podell and colleagues[92] showed that field dependency as measured by echopraxia on manual postures of the ECB was seen in TBI in general and that echopraxia on manual postures is a powerful measure of field dependency. For manual postures, the examiner sits across from the patient and asks him or her to copy various arm and hand positions, making sure that the patient correctly matches the positions of the examiner's right and left sides with the patient's right and left. The patient must be able to mentally manipulate right and left and "reverse" the position to ensure that he or she maintains right and left orientation while not being pulled by the visual stimuli, and mirror what he or she sees (so that the patient's right matches the examiner's left and vice versa). While the initial data are promising, further normative data are required before clinical application of this test can become widespread.

The Delis-Kaplan Executive Function System
The D-KEFS comprises 9 specific tests, which are mostly based on stand-alone tests of executive function. In comparison with stand-alone tests, the D-KEFS is better normed and is better suited to avoid ceiling and floor effects. Several additional quantitative measurements were designed. However, the D-KEFS was not designed to allow for composite score calculation. The 9 independent tests are: The Trail Making Test; The Verbal Fluency Test; Design Fluency; The Color-Word Interference Test, a modification of the Stroop test with addition of Interference/Switching condition; The Sorting Test; The Twenty Questions Test, which resembles the familiar game; The Word Context Test, which involves inferring what a nonsense word means based on clues; The Tower Test; and The Proverb Test, which involves interpreting common and uncommon proverbs and measures the ability to thin.

Actor-centered nature of executive control
Prefrontal cortex is particularly critical for actor-centered decision making. Actor-centered and veridical decision making are based on different mechanisms. Veridical decision making is based on the identification of the correct response (such as, for example, the value of 2 plus 2), which is intrinsic to the external situation and is actor-independent, whereas actor-centered decision making is guided by the actor's priorities. An actor-centered, as opposed to veridical, decision-making process involves relating individual priorities to the parameters of the external situation such as, for example, ordering food in a restaurant.[93]

Because most of the current neuropsychological tests are deterministic and veridical, rigid structure of such tests minimizes their ability to identify the executive function deficit in a clinical evaluation. Even those cognitive tasks that have been traditionally accepted as the "frontal-lobe" tasks (eg, WCST, Category Test, or Stroop test), are quite limited in their ability to elucidate the functions of the frontal lobes, because they are veridical rather than actor-centered. Because the frontal lobes are particularly critical for actor-centered decision making, innovative experimental procedures are required to characterize the contribution of the prefrontal cortex to actor-centered decision making. At present, only very few tests capable of examining adaptive decision making and its impairment exist in clinical neuropsychology. A new generation of tests is needed to measure actor-centered rather than veridical decision making. Two tests, The CBT and The IGT, are among the first steps in this direction.

The Cognitive Bias Task
The CBT[94,95] consists of stimuli characterized along 5 binary variables: color, shape, number, size, and contour. This gradation allows construction of 32 different stimuli. Any 2 stimuli can be compared according to the number of dimensions that they share.

A "similarity index" can be computed, ranging between 5 and 0.The unique feature of the CBT is that it requires that the subject make a response selection based on preference, rather than on any of the external stimulus characteristics or constraints. Original study has demonstrated that CBT is sensitive to the effects of prefrontal lesions, as long as the choice of response is ambiguous and up to the subject, but once the ambiguity is removed, the prefrontal lesion effects disappear.[94] The role played by the prefrontal cortex in the CBT is clearly not in computing the veridical aspects of the task, but in deciding how the inherently ambiguous task should be constrained.

The Iowa Gambling Test

The IGT was originally developed to assess decision making in patients with damage to the ventromedial prefrontal cortex.[87] This test emulates gambling with varied cost versus payoff ratios. Ventromedial prefrontal cortex region of the brain controls aspects of decision making. Bechara and colleagues[96] noted that one factor that was strongly associated with a poor score on the IGT was the inability to maintain employment, which is one of the hallmarks of decision-making impairment in patients with damage to ventromedial prefrontal cortex.

The CBT and the IGT are among the first attempts to develop measures of nonveridical decision making. It is hoped that a whole new generation of neuropsychological tests will emerge, designed to assess various aspects of adaptive decision making.

Working Memory and its Assessment

Over the last few decades, the work by Patricia Goldman-Rakic[72] and Joaquin Fuster[74] helped to clarify the role of the frontal lobes in memory. More specifically, the frontal lobes have been linked with the concept of "working memory." However, the construct of working memory has been somewhat overused. Sometimes it is used interchangeably with the construct of short-term memory. One unique aspect of the concept of working memory is its actor-centered nature—its "what needs to be memorized?" aspect.

In real life, memory recall involves making a decision as to what type of information is useful at the moment, and then selecting this information, when necessary, making a switch from one selection to another. Such decisions require complex neural computations, which are carried out by the frontal lobes. The frontal lobes constantly, and rapidly, "decide" which information is required at which stage of decision making and brings new networks on-line, while letting go of the old ones. Memory based on such a constantly updating selection process guided by the frontal lobes is called working memory.

The main difference between a typical memory test and the way memory is used in real life is that in real life we have to make the decision regarding what to remember, whereas in a typical memory experiment the decision is made for us. This, to a large extent, removes the role of the frontal lobes in experimental memory tasks.

Working memory is among most vulnerable aspects of cognition, and it suffers in a wide range of neurological and psychiatric conditions including TBI. One of the indirect measures of working memory is the semantic clustering index of The California Verbal Learning Test (CVLT).[97] This index provides a measure of the extent to which an individual is capable of independently coming up with a strategy that facilitates the learning of a seemingly large number of unrelated items.

NEUROPSYCHOLOGICAL DEFICITS ASSOCIATED WITH TBI

TBI is associated with a wide range of physiological, behavioral, emotional, and cognitive sequelae. The extent and degree of sequelae varies depending on the severity and location of the injury mitigated by premorbid and post-injury factors and support.

Mild TBI

Acutely, patients can experience a wide range of physiological, sensory, behavioral, emotional, and cognitive deficits.[7] Some combination of concussion-related symptoms such as headache, sensitivity to light and sound, fatigue, dizziness, imbalance, blurred/double vision, emotional lability, and sleep disturbances (too much or too little) are often experienced,[98] but are generally short-lived and resolve over hours to weeks. It is common for acutely concussed patients to have difficulties with thinking, memory, concentration and focus, and fatigue, to often report trouble focusing and paying attention, being forgetful, having trouble with multitasking, feeling tired, and being irritable and short-tempered. Several meta-analyses have demonstrated that these deficits tend to resolve over weeks to months.[99,100] However, some studies have shown small but persistent deficits in some mild TBI patients in speed of processing.[101] The clinical meaningfulness of these findings is unclear.

Fatigue, depression, and anxiety are reported in some mild TBI patients.[7] The extent and duration of the depression is considered complicated and difficult to determine. Issues of a reactive component and neurogenic factors likely interplay with other factors such as pain, work status, litigation status, and premorbid factors.

There exists significant controversy regarding the impact of a positive neuroimaging study on prognosis in patients categorized as mild TBI. Theoretically, the presence of an acute intracranial lesion on neuroimaging would portend a greater degree of injury and concomitant impact on recovery. Earlier studies suggested that patients with a mild TBI and positive finding on neuroimaging performed more like patients with moderate TBI on several neuropsychological tests 1 and 3 months after injury and were more impaired than mild TBI patients with normal neuroimaging.[102–104] Other investigators have reported the same extending to 1 year after injury.[102,103] More recent studies have found similar, but less compelling differences. Iverson[17] found a small to moderate effect size in acute neuropsychological performance (within 2 weeks of injury) between complicated and uncomplicated mild TBI, with minimal difference at 3 months after injury.[24] However, mild TBI patients with positive acute lesions on neuroimaging are at a significantly higher (30%–50%) risk of developing epilepsy,[35,105] which in itself can lead to greater neuropsychological deficits, if not well controlled.

Moderate TBI

Deficits associated with moderate TBI are poorly understood, and the distinction between moderate and severe TBI is blurred. Although individuals enduring a moderate TBI can return to a productive and independent life, they frequently display pervasive, long-term deficits associated with frontal (executive control, behavioral regulation, and working memory) and temporal lobe (learning and memory) functioning, along with depression, anxiety, and emotional dysregulation[7,102,106] that affect daily living and functioning.

Patients with moderate TBI show improvement over the first several months, which tends to plateau within the first year after injury. The ability of moderate TBI patients to return to work is variable. Doctor and colleagues[107] indicated 46% of individuals with moderate TBI (as assessed by GCS) were unemployed 1 year after injury. Similarly, Dikmen and colleagues[108] suggested 45% return to work 6 months after injury whereas about 65% of individuals with moderate TBI have returned to work after 2 years, but often with residual deficits.[7]

Severe TBI

Ten percent or less of the individuals with TBI meets the criteria for severe TBI. Though only a small percentage of all TBI victims, individuals with severe TBI constitute a disproportionate and growing dilemma for society because of the cost and need for extensive rehabilitation and life-long care.[7] Individuals with severe TBI often demonstrate global cognitive, behavioral, and functional deficits even years or decades after the injury.[109] Cognitively, the deficits are pervasive and often severe, with the most profound impairments in the spheres of attention, working memory, learning and memory, and frontal lobe/executive functions.[110] Executive dysfunction often presents as the most debilitating aspect for these patients and can manifest as affective flattening and/or lability, impulsivity/disinhi-bition, amotivation, apathy, poor initiation, impaired planning/organization, and lack of insight. Often, individuals with severe TBI have difficulties with self-regulation, guidance, and awareness of the behavior that interferes with the individual's ability to participate in therapy[111] and return to work.[112] Severe TBI individuals may have trouble regulating their behavior and are prone to greater lability, with outbursts and depression. These patients may be impaired in their ability to detect and correct their own errors in everyday functioning and to use feedback to improve or correct their functioning and behavior. The attentional deficits are extensive and often manifest as poor focus and distractibility, and impaired multitasking to the point of interfering with their ability to work independently[113] or engage in retraining.[114] The memory impairment is characterized by poor acquisition and retrieval,[115] impaired source memory,[116] and typically, but not always, better recognition.[117]

SUMMARY

TBI is a neurological injury that may affect the cognitive, emotional, psychological, and physical functioning of an individual. The clinical neuropsychologist working with TBI patients must take a holistic approach and consider the patient in total, including pre-morbid and post-incident factors, when assessing and treating the patient in order to formulate a comprehensive and accurate picture of the patient that will be used to build an accurate diagnostic impression and guide multiple types of treatment the patient may require. The literature to date indicates a relationship between TBI severity, breadth and severity of neuropsychological deficits, and recovery pattern.

Neuropsychological assessment of executive control/frontal lobe function is of crucial importance in TBI, as the frontal lobes are particularly vulnerable in such an injury. Several neuropsychological tests of executive functions are commonly used and can pick up underlying functional deficits even in the presence of normal neuroimaging. Different tests have their strengths and limitations, which need to be understood in order to quantitate the functional deficit, to correlate the deficit with the clinical presentations, and to properly integrate the findings with the therapeutic plan.

In light of the pervasive nature of the executive deficit, assessment of executive functions is of crucial importance in TBI. Executive control deficits are often multifactorial, and no single-measure executive control function adequately assesses for all of the components. Various tests and batteries are currently available, and it is essential to understand how they are used and interpreted to appropriately apply the findings. When done well, neuropsychological testing is instrumental to understanding brain function and designing interventions that will maximize patient outcomes. Future directions of scientific inquiry in the development of neuropsychological measures of executive functions along the lines of veridical versus adaptive decision-making processes and the "hot" versus "cool" executive processes may further enhance our understanding of executive dysfunction in various neurological and neuropsychiatric conditions, including TBI.

REFERENCES

1. Barth JT, Pliskin N, Axelrod B, et al. Introduction to the NAN 2001 definition of a clinical neuropsychologist. Arch Clin Neuropsychol 2003;18:551–5.
2. Zillmer EA, Spiers MV, Culbertson WC. Principles of neuropsychology. Belmont (CA): Thompson Wadsworth; 2008.
3. Heaton RK, Marcotte TD. Clinical neuropsychological tests and assessment techniques. In: Boller F, Grafman J, Rizzolatti G, editors. Handbook of neuropsychology. Amsterdam: Elsevier Science B. V.; 2000.
4. Rohling ML, Demakis GJ. Failure to replicate or just failure to notice. Does effort still account for more variance in neuropsychological test scores than TBI severity? Clin Neuropsychol 2010;24:119–36.
5. Chaytor N, Temkin N, Machamer J, et al. The ecological validity of neuropsychological assessment and the role of depressive symptoms in moderate to severe traumatic brain injury. J Int Neuropsychol Soc 2007;13:377–85.
6. Asikainen I, Kaste M, Sarnas S. Predicting late outcome for patients with traumatic brain injury referred to a rehabilitation programme: a study of 508 Finnish patients 5 years or more after injury. Brain Inj 1998;12:95–107.
7. Lezak MD, Howieson DB, Loring DW. Neuropsychological assessment. 4th edition. Oxford (UK): Oxford University Press; 2004.
8. Sweeney JE. Nonimpact brain injury: grounds for clinical study of the neuropsychological effects of acceleration forces. Clin Neuropsychol 1992;6:443–57.
9. Gronwall D. Minor head injury. Neuropsychology 1991;5:253–65.
10. Gaultieri R, Cox DR. The delayed neurobehavioral sequelae of traumatic brain injury. Brain Inj 1991;5:219–32.
11. Covassin T, Elbin R, Kontos A, et al. Investigating baseline neurocognitive performance between male and female athletes with a history of multiple concussion. J Neurol Neurosurg Psychiatr 2010;81:597–601.
12. Iverson GL, Brooks BL, Lovell MR, et al. No cumulative effects for one or two previous concussions. Br J Sports Med 2006;40:72–5.
13. Kim E, Lauterbach EC, Reeve A, et al. Neuropsychiatric complications of traumatic brain injury: a critical review of the literature (A report by the ANPA committee on research). J Neuropsychiatry Clin Neurosci 2007;19:106–27.
14. Bombardier CH, Fann JR, Temkin NR, et al. Rates of major depressive disorder and clinical outcomes following traumatic brain injury. J Am Med Assoc 2010; 303:1938–45.
15. Gasquoine PG. Postconcussion symptoms. Neuropsychol Rev 1997;7:77–85.
16. Langenecker SC, Lee HJ, Bieliauskas LA. Neuropsychology of depression and related mood disorders. In: Grant I, Adams K, editors. Neuropsychological assessment of neuropsychiatric and neuromedical disorders. Oxford (UK): University Press; 2009. p. 523–59.
17. Iverson GL. Complicated vs. uncomplicated mild traumatic brain injury: acute neuropsychological outcome. Brain Inj 2006;20:1335–44.
18. Vasterlin JJ, Bailey K, Constans JI, et al. Attention and memory dysfunction in posttraumatic stress disorder. Neuropsychology 1998;12:125–33.
19. Danckwerts A, Leathem J. Questioning the link between PTSD and cognitive dysfunction. Neuropsychol Rev 2003;13:221–35.
20. Greiffenstein M, Baker W. Validity testing in dually diagnosed post-traumatic stress disorder and mild closed head injury. Clin Neuropsychol 2008;22:565–82.
21. Mooney G, Speed J. The association between mild traumatic brain injury and psychiatric conditions. Brain Injury 2001;15:865–77.

22. Rourke SB, Grant I. The neurobehavioral correlates of alcoholism. In: Grant I, Adams K, editors. Neuropsychological assessment of neuropsychiatric and neuromedical disorders. Oxford (UK): University Press; 2009. p. 398–454.

23. Gonzalez R, Vassileva J, Scott JC. Neuropsychological consequences of drug abuse. In: Grant I, Adams K, editors. Neuropsychological assessment of neuropsychiatric and neuromedical disorders. Oxford (UK): University Press; 2009. p. 455–79.

24. Lange RT, Iverson GL, Franzen MD. Comparability of neuropsychological test profiles in patients with chronic substance abuse and mild traumatic brain injury. Clin Neuropsychol 2008;22:209–27.

25. Larrabee GJ. Neuropsychology in personal injury litigation. J Clin Exp Neuropsychol 2000;22:702–7.

26. Green P, Rohling ML, Lees-Haley PR, et al. Effort has a greater effect on test scores than severe brain injury in compensation claimants. Brain Inj 2001;15: 1045–60.

27. Moore BA, Donders J. Predictors of invalid neuropsychological test performance after traumatic brain injury. Brain Inj 2004;18:975–84.

28. Nampiaparampil DE. Prevalence of chronic pain after traumatic brain injury. J Am Med Assoc 2008;300:711–9.

29. Hart RP, Martelli MF, Zasler ND. Chronic pain and neuropsychological functioning. Neuropsychol Rev 2000;10:131–49.

30. Sjogren P, Thomsen AB, Olsen AK. Impaired neuropsychological performance in chronic nonmalignant pain patients receiving long-term oral opioid therapy. J Pain Symptom Manage 2000;19:100–8.

31. Lees-Haley PR. Toxic mold and mycotoxins in neurotoxicity cases: Stachybotrys, fusarium, trichoderma, aspergillus, penicillin, cladosporium, alternaria, trichothecenes. Psychol Rep 2003;93:561–84.

32. Greiffenstein MF. Basics of forensic neuropsychology. In: Morgan JE, Ricker JH, editors. Textbook of Clinical Neuropsychology. New York: Taylor & Francis; 2008. p. 905–41.

33. Boone KB, Lu P. Noncredible cognitive performance in the context of severe brain injury. Clin Neuropsychol 2003;17(2):244.

34. Rogers R. Models of feigned illness. Prof Psychol Res Pr 1990;21:182–8.

35. Carroll LJ, Cassidy JD, Peloso PM, et al. Prognosis for mild traumatic brain injury: results of the WHO collaborating centre task force on mild traumatic brain injury. J Rehabil Med 2004;43(Suppl):84–105.

36. Harris I, Mulford J, Solomon M, et al. Association between compensation status and outcome after surgery: a meta-analysis. J Am Med Assoc 2005;293(13): 1644–52.

37. Pobereskin LH. Whiplash following rear end collisions: a prospective cohort study. J Neurol Neurosurg Psychiatry 2005;76(8):1146–51.

38. Mittenburg W, Aguila-Puentes G, Patton C, et al. Neuropsychological profiling of symptom exaggeration and malingering. J Forensic Neuropsychol 2002;3: 227–40.

39. Carroll S, Abrahmse A, Vaiana M. The costs of excess medical claims for automobile personal injuries. Santa Monica (CA): RAND; 1995.

40. Larrabee GJ. Detection of malingering using atypical performance patterns on standard neuropsychological test. Clin Neuropsychol 2003;17:410–25.

41. Belanger HG, Curtiss G, Demery JA, et al. Factors moderating neuropsychological outcomes following mild traumatic brain injury: a meta-analysis. J Int Neuropsychol Soc 2005;11(3):215–27.

42. Paniak C, Reynolds S, Toller-Lobe G, et al. A longitudinal study of the relationship between financial compensation and symptoms after treated mild traumatic brain injury. J Clin Exp Neuropsychol 2002;24(2):187–93.
43. Tsaousides T, Gordon WA. Cognitive rehabilitation following traumatic brain injury: assessment to treatment. Mt Sinai J Med 2009;76:173–81.
44. Ryu WH, Cullen NK, Bayley MT. Early neuropsychological tests as correlates of productivity 1 year after traumatic brain injury: a preliminary matched case-control study. Int J Rehabil Res 2010;33:84–7.
45. Atchison TB, Sander AM, Struchen MA, et al. Relationship between neuropsychological test performance and productivity at 1-year following traumatic brain injury. Clin Neuropsychol 2004;18:248–65.
46. Levin HS, O'Donnell VM, Grossman RG. The Galveston Orientation and Amnesia Test. a practical scale to assess cognition after head injury. J Nerv Ment Dis 1979;167:675–84.
47. Ellenburg JH, Levin HS, Saydjari C. Posttraumatic amnesia as a predictor of outcome after severe closed head injury. Arch Neurol 1996;53:782–91.
48. Kane R. Standardized and flexible batteries in neuropsychology: an assessment update. Neuropsychol Rev 1991;2:281–339.
49. Incagnoli T, Goldstein G, Golden CJ, editors. Neuropsychological test batteries. New York: Plenum; 1986.
50. Heaton RK, Pendleton MG. Use of neuropsychological tests to predict adult patient's everyday functioning. J Consult Clin Psychol 1981;49:807–21.
51. Parsons OA. Overview of the Halstead-Reitan battery. In: Incagnoli T, Goldstein G, Golden C, editors. Clinical applications of neuropsychological test batteries. New York: Plenum; 1986. p. 155–89.
52. Reitan RM, Wolfson D. The Halstead-Reitan neuropsychological test battery. Tempe (AZ): Neuropsychology Press; 1985.
53. Goodglass H. The flexible battery. In: Incagnoli T, Goldstein G, Golden CJ, editors. neuropsychological assessment. New York: Plenum; 1986. p. 121–31.
54. Schear JM. Neuropsychological assessment of the elderly in clinical practice. In: Logue PE, Schear JM, editors. Clinical neuropsychology: a multidisciplinary approach. Springfield (IL): Charles C Thomas; 1984. p. 199–236.
55. Russell EW. Theory and development of pattern analysis methods related to the Halstead-Reitan battery. In: Logue PE, Schear JM, editors. Clinical neuropsychology: a multidisciplinary approach. Springfield (IL): Charles C Thomas; 1984. p. 50–62.
56. Kaplan E. Process and achievement revisited. In: Wapner S, Kaplan B, editors. Towards a holistic developmental psychology. Hillsdale (NJ): Lawrence Erlbaum Associates; 1983. p. 143–56.
57. Tarter RE, Edwards KL. Neuropsychological batteries. In: Incagnoli T, Goldstein G, Golden CJ, editors. Clinical application of neuropsychological test batteries. New York: Plenum; 1986. p. 135–52.
58. La Rue A, et al. Aging and neuropsychological assessment. New York: Plenum; 1992.
59. Heaton RK, Grant I, Matthews CG. Comprehensive norms for an expanded Halstead-Reitan battery. Odessa (FL): Psychological Assessment Resources; 1991.
60. Greiffenstein MF, Baker WJ, Johnson-Greene D. Actual versus self-reported scholastic achievement of litigating post-concussion and severe closed head injury claimants. Psychol Assess 2002;14:202–8.

61. Greiffenstein MF, Baker WJ. Premorbid clues? preinjury scholastic performance and present neuropsychological functioning in late postconcussion syndrome. Clin Neuropsychol 2003;17:561–73.

62. Johnstone B, Callahan CD, Kaplia CJ, et al. The comparability of the WRAT-R reading test and NAART as estimates of premorbid intelligence in neurologically impaired patients. Arch Clin Neuropsychol 1996;11:513–9.

63. Benton AL, Hamsher K, Varney N, et al. Contributions to neuropsychological assessment: a clinical manual. New York: Oxford University Press; 1983.

64. Wechsler D. Wechsler adult intelligence scale—III. San Antonio (TX): The Psychological Corporation; 1997.

65. Wechsler D. Wechsler memory scale. third edition manual. San Antonio (TX): The Psychological Corporation; 1997.

66. Goldberg E, Bilder RM. The frontal lobes and hierarchical organization of cognitive control. In: Perecman E, editor. The frontal lobes revisited. New York: IRBN Press; 1987. p. 159–87.

67. Wheeler MA, Stuss DT, Tulving E. Toward a theory of episodic memory: the frontal lobes and autonoetic consciousness. Psychol Bull 1997;121:331–54.

68. Goldberg E. Introduction: the frontal lobes in neurological and psychiatric conditions. Neuropsychiatry Neuropsychol Behav Neurol 1992;5(4):231–2.

69. Goldberg E, Bougakov D. Novel approaches to the diagnosis and treatment of frontal lobe dysfunction. In: Christensen A-L, Uzzel BP, editors. International handbook of neuropsychological rehabilitation. New York: Kluwer Academic/Plenum Publishers; 2000. p. 93–112.

70. Deutsch G, Eisenberg HM. Frontal blood flow changes in recovery from coma. J Cereb Blood Flow Metab 1987;7(1):29–34.

71. Luria AR. Higher cortical functions in man. New York: Basic Books; 1966.

72. Goldman-Rakic PS. Circuitry of primate prefrontal cortex and regulation of behavior by representational memory. In: Plum F, editor. Handbook of physiology: nervous system, higher functions of the brain (part 1), vol. 5. 5th edition. Bethesda (MD): American Physiological Association; 1987. p. 373–417.

73. Milner B. Some cognitive effects of frontal lobe lesion in man. Philos Trans R Soc Lond 1982;298:211–26.

74. Fuster J. The prefrontal cortex. 4th edition. London, England: Academic Press; 2008.

75. Shallice T. Specific impairments of planning. Philos Trans R Soc Lond B Biol Sci 1982;298(1089):199–209.

76. Grant DA, Berg EA. A behavioral analysis of degree of reinforcement and ease of shifting to new responses in a Weigl-type card-sorting problem. J Exp Psychol 1948;38:404–11.

77. Halstead W, Settlage P. Grouping behavior of normal persons and of persons with lesions of the brain: further analysis. Arch Neurol Psychiatry 1943;49(4): 489–506.

78. Stroop JR. Studies of interference in serial verbal reactions. J Exp Psychol 1935; 18:643–62.

79. Jensen AR, Rohwer WD Jr. The Stroop color-word test: a review. Acta Psychol (Amst) 1966;25(1):36–93.

80. Eriksen BA, Eriksen CW. Effects of noise letters upon the identification of a target letter in a nonsearch task. Percept Psychophys 1974;16:143–9.

81. Eriksen CW, Schultz DW. Information processing in visual search: A continuous flow conception and experimental results. Percept Psychophys 1979;25(4): 249–63.

82. Dyer FN, Severance LJ. Stroop interference with successive presentations of separate incongruent words and colors. J Exp Psychol 1973;98(2):438–9.

83. Stuss DT, Floden D, Alexander MP, et al. Stroop performance in focal lesion patients: dissociation of processes and frontal lobe lesion location. Neuropsychologia 2001;39(8):771–86.

84. Halterman Charlene I, Langan Jeanne, Drew Anthony, et al. Tracking the recovery of visuospatial attention deficits in mild traumatic brain injury. Brain 2006;129(3):747–53.

85. Hongwanishkul D, Happaney KR, Lee W, et al. Hot and cool executive function: age-related changes and individual differences. Dev Neuropsychol 2005;28: 617–44.

86. Zelazo PD, Cunningham W. Executive function: mechanisms underlying emotion regulation. In: Gross J, editor. Handbook of emotion regulation. New York: Guilford; 2007. p. 135–58.

87. Bechara A, Damasio AR, Damasio H, et al. Insensitivity to future consequences following damage to human prefrontal cortex. Cognition 1994;50(1–3):7–15.

88. Kerr A, Zelazo PD. Development of "hot" executive function: the children's gambling task. Brain Cogn 2004;55:148–57.

89. Delis D, Kaplan E, Kramer J. Delis-Kaplan executive function scale. San Antonio (TX): Psychological Corporation; 2001.

90. Goldberg E, Podell K, Bilder R, et al. The executive control battery. Australia: Psych Press; 2000.

91. Podell K, Lovell M. The manual postures test: a clinically useful measure of echopraxia. Paper presented at the International Neuropsychological Society 27th Annual Meeting. Boston (MA), 1999.

92. Podell K, Wisniewski K, Lovell M. The assessment of echopraxia as a component of executive control deficit in traumatic brain injury. Poster presented at the 10th annual Rotman Research Institute Conference. Toronto, Canada, 1999.

93. Goldberg E, Podell K. Adaptive decision making, ecological validity, and the frontal lobes. J Clin Exp Neuropsychol 2000;22:56–68.

94. Goldberg E, Harner R, Lovell M, et al. Cognitive bias, functional cortical geometry, and the frontal lobes: laterality, sex, and handedness. J Cogn Neurosci 1994;6(3):276–96.

95. Podell K, Lovell M, Zimmerman M, et al. The cognitive bias task and lateralized frontal lobe functions in males. J Neuropsychiatry Clin Neurosci 1995;7(4): 491–501.

96. Bechara A, Dolan S, Denburg N, et al. Decision-making deficits, linked to a dysfunctional ventromedial prefrontal cortex, revealed in alcohol and stimulant abusers. Neuropsychologia 2001;39(4):376–89.

97. Delis D, Kaplan E, Kramer J, et al. California verbal learning test—second edition (CVLT-II). San Antonio (TX): Psychological Corporation; 2000.

98. Bazarian JJ, Zhong J, Blyth B, et al. Diffusion tensor imaging detects clinically important axonal damage after mild traumatic brain injury: a pilot study. J Neurotrauma 2007;24:1447–59.

99. Larrabee GJ. Neuropsychological outcome, post concussion symptoms, and forensic considerations in mild closed head trauma. Semin Clin Neuropsychiatry 1997;2(3):196–206.

100. Schretlen DJ, Shapiro AM. A quantitative review of the effects of traumatic brain injury on cognitive functioning. Int Rev Psychiatry 2003;15(4):341–9.

101. Bernstein DM. Information processing difficulty long after self-reported concussion. J Int Neuropsychol Soc 2002;8:673–82.

102. Kasluba S, Hanks RA, Casey JE, et al. Neuropsychologic and functional outcome after complicated mild traumatic brain injury. Arch Phys Med Rehabil 2008;89:904–11.
103. Borgaro SR, Prigatano GP, Kwasnica C, et al. Cognitive and affective sequelae in complicated and uncomplicated mild traumatic brain injury. Brain Inj 2003;17: 189–98.
104. Kurca E, Sivák S, Kucera P. Impaired cognitive functions in mild traumatic brain injury patients with normal and pathologic magnetic resonance imaging. Neuroradiology 2006;48:661–9.
105. Diaz-Arrastia R, Agostini MA, Madden CJ, et al. Posttraumatic epilepsy: the endophenotypes of a human model of epileptogenesis. Epilepsia 2009;50:14–20.
106. Iverson GL. Outcome from mild traumatic brain injury. Curr Opin Psychiatry 2005;18:301–17.
107. Doctor JN, Castro J, Temkin NR, et al. Worker's risk of unemployment after traumatic brain injury: a normed comparison. J Int Neuropsychol Soc 2005;11: 747–52.
108. Dikmen SS, Temkin NR, Machamer JE, et al. Employment following traumatic brain injury. Arch Neurol 1994;51:177–86.
109. Hoofien D, Gilboa A, Vakil E, et al. Traumatic brain injury (TBI) 10–20 years later: a comprehensive approach to culture and cognition. Brain Inj 2001;15:189–209.
110. Millis SR, Rosenthal M, Novack TA, et al. Long-term neuropsychological outcome after traumatic brain injury. J Head Trauma Rehabil 2001;16:343–55.
111. Ben-Yishay Y, Diller L. Cognitive remediation in traumatic brain injury: updates and issues. Arch Phys Med Rehabil 1993;74:204–13.
112. Sherer M, Bergloff P, Levin E, et al. Impaired awareness and employment outcome after traumatic brain injury. J Head Trauma Rehabil 1998;13:52–61.
113. Whyte J, Schuster K, Polansky M, et al. Frequency and duration of inattentive behavior after traumatic brain injury: Effects of distraction, task, and practice. J Int Neuropsychol Soc 2000;6:1–11.
114. Wood RL. Disorders of attention and their treatment in traumatic brain injury rehabilitation. In: Bigler ED, editor. Traumatic brain injury. Austin (TX): Pro-Ed; 1990. p. 121–39.
115. Brooks J, Hosie J, Bond MR. Cognitive sequelae of severe head injury in relation to Glasgow outcome scale. J Neurol Neurosurg Psychiatry 1986;49:549–53.
116. Crosson B, Novack TA, Trenerry MR, et al. Differentiation of verbal memory deficits in blunt head injury using the recognition trial of the California verbal learning tests: an exploratory study. Clin Neuropsychol 1989;3:29–44.
117. Spikman JM, Berg IJ, Deelman BG. Spared recognition capacity in elderly and closed-head-injury subjects with clinical memory deficits. J Clin Exp Neuropsychol 1995;17:29–34.

Rehabilitation of Traumatic Brain Injury

Jaime M. Levine, DO*, Steven R. Flanagan, MD

KEYWORDS

- Traumatic brain injury • Rehabilitation
- Multidisciplinary approach • Cognitive impairments

DEFINITION AND REHABILITATION VENUE

Neurorehabilitation is a general term used to describe the rehabilitation of people who have functional deficits resulting from a disease or injury to the central nervous system (CNS). Although the causes of CNS dysfunction are vast in number and include ischemia, infection, neoplasm, hypoxia, and trauma, this article focuses on the neurorehabilitation of people who have sustained a traumatic brain injury (TBI). TBI causes many problems common to other conditions requiring rehabilitation, such as paresis and associated impairments in mobility and the ability to safely perform activities of daily living (ADL). However, it also causes cognitive and behavioral impairments that are often the primary barrier to successful community reintegration, and requires a thoughtful and well-coordinated assessment and treatment approach to achieve the most desirable outcomes. TBI is also associated with several unique comorbidities that require careful attention to properly diagnose and treat.

There are various settings where TBI rehabilitation can be provided, including acute facilities, subacute facilities, home, and outpatient settings. The appropriate location is dependent on several factors, including the severity of injury and associated physical, cognitive, and behavioral impairments, the need for ongoing medical oversight, and time after injury. Once a person with TBI has been medically stabilized post trauma and no longer requires continual intensive care treatments, but has persistent TBI-related functional impairments, transfer to a rehabilitation setting should be considered. Acute inpatient rehabilitation typically occurs in specialized brain injury units situated within a hospital or a freestanding facility. Certain admission criteria must be met before acceptance to an acute rehabilitation unit including:

- Medical complexity that requires around-the-clock physician presence and specialized rehabilitative nursing expertise

Rusk Institute of Rehabilitation Medicine, New York University School of Medicine, New York, NY, USA
* Corresponding author. 400 East 34 Street, Room 119, New York, NY 10016.
E-mail address: jaime.levine@nyumc.org

Psychiatr Clin N Am 33 (2010) 877–891
doi:10.1016/j.psc.2010.09.001
0193-953X/10/$ – see front matter © 2010 Elsevier Inc. All rights reserved.

psych.theclinics.com

- Reasonable expectation for functional improvement and discharge to the community within a reasonable period of time
- Functional deficits requiring at least 3 hours of specialized rehabilitation treatment.

Individuals who do not meet these criteria but who cannot return to their home because of persistent TBI-related functional impairments should be considered for subacute rehabilitation, which provides less intensive medical, nursing, and rehabilitation interventions in long-term care facilities. Home-based rehabilitation is provided to those individuals who no longer require close medical oversight or daily therapy. Home therapy is typically reserved for those people who are homebound and cannot travel to outpatient rehabilitation settings. Outpatient therapy is provided to those people who can travel outside their home on a regular basis and have ongoing rehabilitation needs.

Regardless of the setting, rehabilitation is provided in an interdisciplinary manner by a specialized team of health care providers, the patient, and his or her loved ones. The interdisciplinary model takes advantage of each member's unique knowledge and expertise while the entire team works collaboratively to address impairments that cut across multiple disciplines. The team is usually led by a physiatrist, a physician with specialized training in physical medicine and rehabilitation who oversees and coordinates the care provided by other team members and medical specialists. Other members of the interdisciplinary team are included based on the individual needs of the patient and typically include a physical therapist, occupational therapist, speech-language pathologist, recreation therapist, neuropsychologist, rehabilitation nurse, social worker, vocational counselor, and case manager, and invariably the patient and his or her loved ones.

ACUTE INPATIENT REHABILITATION

Rehabilitation interventions ideally begin when a patient is still on an acute neurosurgical or trauma service with the goals of maintaining joint and limb flexibility, skin integrity, pulmonary health, and ability to tolerate sitting in and out of bed. Once sufficient medical stability has been achieved and the primary focus of care becomes restoration of lost functional skills, more intensive rehabilitation ensues in a specialized brain injury unit. The unit is ideally designed to accommodate the unique needs of people with TBI that account for their physical, cognitive, and behavioral problems. The physiatrist assesses the patient's medical and functional status at the time of admission and writes specific orders for other team members, indicating precautions that need to be considered during treatment. Each health care provider assigned to the team assesses the patient and, along with the patient and loved ones, establishes a series of goals to achieve during treatment.

Communication among team members occurs on a daily basis, typically during bedside patient rounds that should include the physician, rehabilitation nurse, and therapy representative. More formal weekly patient evaluation conferences are also held. The conference is lead by the physiatrist who provides medical updates while other team members detail the progress made toward previously established short- and long-term goals, which may need to be modified based on the patient's course of recovery. Barriers to community discharge are also discussed with changes in treatment plans made as needed. A plan to ensure a safe discharge to the community is developed, including continued rehabilitation and nursing services, follow-up medical care, and provision of necessary equipment, such as walking aids and bathroom safety devices. If discharge to the community becomes impractical, plans are made to transfer the patient to another level of care, typically subacute rehabilitation. It is important that although communication is an invaluable component of successful rehabilitation, it is not a substitute for first-hand observation; physiatrists should regularly observe therapy sessions to directly monitor their patients' performances. Likewise, nursing and therapy staff need to attend daily bedside rounds with the physician to maintain their awareness of all medical issues pertinent to their patient, and incorporate the necessary precautions as directed by the physiatrist.

Following each evaluation conference, family meetings are scheduled to communicate updates and review discharge plans with loved ones, as well as for the family to share their thoughts regarding the recovery process and future needs. Although this meeting occurs regularly throughout the inpatient process, it is usually brief but highly productive, as it helps to secure a thoughtful consensus regarding medical management, discharge destination, and caregiver designation.

Following discharge to the community, each patient should be scheduled to follow-up with their physiatrist within 6 weeks, or sooner if there is a time-sensitive medical issue that requires earlier attention. With acute rehabilitation lengths of stay becoming shorter, this office visit is increasingly becoming an important opportunity to modulate neuropharmacological agents and to follow up on ongoing medical issues. This office visit serves multiple important purposes and helps to ensure a smooth reentry into the community. A careful medication review should be conducted, with careful attention paid to any psychoactive drugs. Patients should have initiated either home-based or outpatient therapy by this time, which is a good opportunity to review short-term and long-term goals. Resumption of driving is another important topic that should be addressed at this or a later visit as deemed appropriate. Depending on the patient's functional status, it is appropriate to seek feedback from his or her therapy team regarding readiness for a dedicated driving retraining program. The therapy team is also an excellent resource for guidance regarding vocational training when appropriate.

Restriction on the length of impatient rehabilitation imposed by third-party payers represents a significant challenge in providing sufficient care to people with TBI. From 2000 to 2007, the mean acute rehabilitation length of stay among brain-injured patients decreased from 22.7 ($\pm$ 20.5) to 16.6 ($\pm$ 14.8) days.[1] The Prospective Payment System, enacted by the Commission on Medicare and Medicaid Services (CMS), imposed a significant financial barrier to providing sufficient inpatient rehabilitation services to Medicare beneficiaries, which may further adversely affect length of stay.[2]

SPECIAL CONSIDERATIONS
Therapy and Medical Test Scheduling

Cognitive impairments constitute one of the main challenges in TBI rehabilitation. New learning, which is often severely impaired following TBI, is essential to secure the skills necessary to achieve independence in mobility and ADL. To help promote the consolidation of new learning, a unit-wide schedule must be created that allocates ample rest time between therapy sessions. While actual physical practice is needed to learn a specific motor skill, sleep and rest play an important role in consolidating the memory of that task[3,4]; this helps to induce neuronal changes that strengthen and stabilize the new skill.[5] In addition to creating an overnight environment conducive to sleep, 60 to 90 minutes of designated rest during the mid-day hours enhances this process. Visitors need to be advised of the importance of this rest time so that they do not inadvertently interfere with the rehabilitation process. This problem may be best addressed by developing strategic visiting hours for each patient that maximizes family involvement and patient recovery while minimizing disruptions in necessary care.

In addition to a unit-wide schedule, individual therapy schedules are tailored to the medical needs and tolerance of each patient. For example, while all patients in an acute inpatient rehabilitation environment participate in a minimum of 3 hours of daily therapy, some will tolerate 3 1-hour blocks whereas others with poor endurance or impaired concentration will have their needs best met with shorter sessions scattered throughout the day. Medical tests or procedures performed off the rehabilitation unit should be scheduled to minimize disruption of the patient's therapy and rest periods. Fatigue-inducing treatments, such as hemodialysis or chemotherapy, should be scheduled following the completion of daily therapy.

Maximizing Safety

Creating a safe environment is a paramount concern during inpatient rehabilitation. The risk of patients falling is great, and their sequelae potentially catastrophic. Numerous factors account for this risk in the brain-injured patient population, including:

- Neurological problems such as paresis, impaired balance, and altered proprioceptive and visuospatial skills[6]
- The unfamiliar physical environment to a cognitively impaired person that represents a deviation from their familiar surroundings
- Impulsivity and poor awareness of deficits
- Cognitive impairments, agitation, and behavioral dysregulation that make it difficult to teach compensatory safety strategies.[7]

Fall prevention is an interdisciplinary effort and is tailored to best match a patient's needs. Interventions often include careful medication monitoring, environmental modifications, balance and strengthening programs, toileting schedules, and bed alarms that address specific risk factors associated with falls.[8] Judicial use of physical restraints can also be used to prevent falls, but acknowledging their use is controversial. When implementing a restraint in this setting, it is essential that other less restrictive interventions have been used and found to be ineffective. The use of a specific restraint is of paramount importance to maximize participation in rehabilitation while enhancing patient safety. For instance, restricting access to a gastrostomy tube by using an abdominal binder is typically preferred to physically restraining an arm or hand. Patient restraints should be reviewed daily by all team members to ensure that the least restrictive and most appropriate means are chosen for that given day. Educating families on the use of restraints is important to ensure compliance and to earn their trust. Elopement is also a frequent concern, as many patients have minimally impaired mobility skills yet significant cognitive impairments that restrict their awareness of safety concerns. This problem may be addressed by providing continual direct patient observation, exit alarm systems, or an exit off the unit equipped with a locking mechanism.

SPECIFIC TBI-RELATED CONDITIONS
Fatigue/Sleep Disturbance

Fatigue is among the most pervasive symptoms after TBI, and occurs at a greater frequency than that in the general population.[9,10] Fatigue is a frequent barrier to successful rehabilitation, as it can shorten and decrease the efficiency of therapy sessions. It is important to address fatigue as part of the admission workup, monitor for signs of fatigue throughout the rehabilitation course, and employ appropriate treatments to address it both pharmacologically and through behavioral modification.

There is no universally accepted definition of fatigue, but many sources describe it as a subjective sense of overwhelming tiredness, lack of energy, and exhaustion. A general distinction is made between central and peripheral fatigue, describing the former as difficulty initiating or sustaining mental or physical tasks in the absence of motor impairments and the latter as musculoskeletal symptoms that affect mobility or the ability to perform ADL. Although peripheral fatigue is common in this population because of motor and musculoskeletal impairments, central fatigue is often more debilitating because it compromises the degree of mental effort and sustained attention available for participation in therapies meant to target both cognitive and physical deficits. It is also important to determine whether the fatigue is primary to the TBI or secondary to another condition, such as depression, pain, sleep disorders, or neuroendocrine abnormalities, which have all been associated with fatigue after TBI.[10,11]

TBI-related fatigue can be treated in a number of ways, including patient and caregiver education, behavioral modification, exercise, and/or pharmacological interventions. Patients should be instructed to tailor physical activities to prevent exhaustion, limit exercise to the morning and afternoon hours to prevent insomnia, and schedule periodic rest breaks throughout the day as needed. Multiple classes of drugs have been anecdotally reported to reduce fatigue, although no clear guidelines or treatment standards exist to date for treating this problem. Agents commonly used to directly ameliorate symptoms of fatigue in the TBI population include neurostimulants, dopaminergic agonists, and antidepressants.

It is well known that sleep patterns commonly become distorted after TBI.[12,13] Therefore, it is often difficult to distinguish central fatigue from that caused by a comorbid sleep disorder. The incidence of sleep disturbances among hospitalized TBI patients can be as high as 36%, manifested most often as a disorder of initiating and/or maintaining sleep.[14] Studies have shown that these patients have decreased rapid-eye-movement and slow-wave sleep, as well an increase in the number of nighttime awakenings.[14] Reports have also shown that brain injury contributes to a shortening of the total sleep time and the disappearance of deep sleep,[15] all potentially exacerbating excessive daytime somnolence.

Treatment options for sleep disorders are extensive and tailored to the specific nature of the disturbance. In each case both pharmacologic and nonpharmacologic treatments should be considered. Nonpharmacologic options, or sleep hygiene techniques, should be adopted and include limitation of caffeine consumption, retiring and awaking at consistent times daily, and removing the clock from view while in bed to reduce anxiety regarding the need to get to sleep. People should be instructed to limit the time they try to get to sleep to 30 to 40 minutes, initiating nonstimulating activities outside of bed for a period of time before attempting sleep again, as well as considering sleeping in other locations.

Pharmacologic options may be considered once sleep hygiene measures have been implemented, and include melatonin receptor agonists, certain antidepressants, sedatives/hypnotics, and antiepileptics. However, sleep-inducing agents must be used with great care in this population because they can potentially worsen cognitive skills, increase the risk of falling, or cause other unwanted side effects.[16] For example, the atypical antidepressant trazodone, which is commonly used to treat sleep-onset disorders in this population, can potentially cause hypotension, blurry vision, and dizziness as well as dry mouth, headache, and nausea.[17] In addition, the newer, non-benzodiazepine sedative hypnotics such as zolpidem, zopiclone, and eszopiclone, while causing less daytime somnolence and fewer withdrawal symptoms than their benzodiazepine counterparts,[18] still have the potential to cause unwanted cognitive effects while the drug is active, and should be used with caution in the TBI population.

Autonomic Instability

Autonomic instability, including intermittent tachycardia, diaphoresis, hypertension, and hyperthermia, is a common complication following severe brain injury. The term paroxysmal autonomic instability with dystonia (PAID) has been proposed to capture the main features of this syndrome.[19] Although PAID has been referred to by various names, including paroxysmal sympathetic storms,[20] dysautonomia,[21] and autonomic dysfunction syndrome,[22] the commonality in features indicates that they all refer to the same phenomenon.

PAID has been recognized in both children and adults, and often causes considerable concern in caregivers because it mimics other life-threatening conditions such as neuroleptic malignant syndrome, sepsis, and malignant hyperthermia. As PAID is a diagnosis of exclusion, inquiries must be made into these other possible causes, though a careful assessment and rapid diagnosis can avoid time-consuming and expensive workups and avoid unnecessary treatments. Although there is no specific workup to diagnose PAID, elevated catecholamine levels in the right context is considered supportive of the diagnosis.[23]

The various treatments for PAID are geared toward its individual components. For example, the nonselective β-blocker propranolol, which is a mainstay of treatment for PAID,[23] ameliorates sympathetic excitation, which if left untreated results in tachycardia and hypertension. Dantrolene is used because of its muscle relaxant and antipyrexic effects. Clonidine, which is often used in this setting, exerts its blood pressure–lowering effects through α2-agonism, and also has sedating properties. The dopamine agonist bromocriptine is used in the treatment of PAID, although its mechanism of effectiveness in this setting is poorly understood. Its use for this indication is based on the similarities between PAID and neuroleptic malignant syndrome, which is caused by a dopamine blockade.[24] Other commonly used agents to treat the components of PAID include lorazepam, which is used for its anxiolytic, muscle-relaxing, and sedating effects, and morphine, because it induces some degree of respiratory depression and bradycardia, thus countering tachypnea and tachycardia. The analgesic property of morphine is also useful in treating painful dystonia.[19]

Cognitive Impairments

Cognitive impairments are extremely pervasive following TBI, and represent a significant barrier to successful reintegration to the patient's community and participation in desired societal roles. Common impairments encountered include, but are not limited to problems with various aspects of memory, learning, attention/concentration, mental processing speed, executive skills, and awareness of impairments. Clinical neuropsychologists are professionals who have special expertise in the area of brain-behavior relationships, and are integrally involved in the identification of specific cognitive impairments and development of individualized treatments and strategies to ameliorate their impact on daily function. However, given the pervasive nature of cognitive impairments, all members of the team must adapt to the specific patterns of cognitive weakness and relatively preserved strengths of each individual patient to effectively tailor a successful rehabilitation program. Neuropsychological testing that details a patient's relative strengths and weakness is an important assessment tool that helps guide the process of cognitive therapy. Limited testing is typically conducted during acute inpatient rehabilitation to quickly identify areas that require immediate intervention. Comprehensive testing is typically reserved after acute inpatient discharge for several reasons, including the rapid rate of cognitive change acutely following TBI. Also, a complete neuropsychological battery is very time consuming, which would use a disproportionate amount of time during what has become a very contracted period allocated for acute inpatient rehabilitation. Formally reassessing cognitive skills periodically is an effective means to monitor the course of recovery and the effectiveness of rehabilitation interventions, acknowledging that sufficient time needs to pass between testing to avoid practice effects and inaccurate results.

Cognitive therapy is often supplemented by medications that have been shown to enhance various cognitive skills. While a comprehensive review here is not practical, it is widely accepted that various drugs that impact specific neurotransmitter systems can improve cognitive skills. Catecholaminergic agonists such as methylphenidate have been thought to improve various aspects of attention,[25] whereas others such as bromocriptine have been suggested to demonstrate improvement in executive skills.[26] Acetylcholine agonists have been shown to improve memory and attention in specific individuals after TBI,[27] noting that people with more impaired skills seem to benefit most.[28] It must be noted, however, that standards regarding the use of medications to improve cognitive skills after TBI have not been established and that their use for such remains off-label.

Once discharged to the community, patients often benefit from continued neuropsychological support. Patients and their family members often realize the full extent of the cognitive and behavioral deficits once they are outside of the sheltered hospital environment, and as this awareness grows it is common to have difficulty adjusting to community living. One's role in the family unit may change, and this can alter the entire family dynamic. Neuropsychologists along with other team members often lead support groups for families, and become important sources of information and counsel.

Agitation

Agitation following TBI is one of the most concerning and anxiety-producing problems faced by health care providers and family members. There are many definitions of TBI-related agitation that encompass a wide variety of nonadaptive behaviors, such as restlessness, impulsivity, uneasiness, edginess, distractibility, and fidgety behavior to more overt symptoms of physical and verbal aggression that often interfere with participation in the rehabilitation process, provision of care, and societal roles. However, agitation may be best defined and distinguished from other related terms or abnormalities of brain function as:

> ...a subtype of delirium unique to survivors of TBI in which the survivor is in the state of post-traumatic amnesia and there are excesses of behavior that include the combination of aggression, akathisia, disinhibition, and/or emotional lability.[29]

Management of agitation depends on an assessment of multiple variables, including patient location, medical status, and the intensity and potential consequences of the undesired behavior. For example, immediate measures such as pharmacological sedation or physical restraints may be indicated when a physically aggressive patient immediately threatens the safety of self, staff, or family members. Conversely, restlessness manifested as continuous walking may not require intervention other than close supervision to prevent elopement of a confused patient. Ideally, it is best to proactively inhibit the development of agitation whenever feasible, rather than reacting to it once it manifests. For example, staff and families should limit excessive stimulation during the early phases of recovery when patients cannot effectively filter competing environmental noise. Therapy sessions should be provided in quiet settings with treatment interventions tailored to promote recovery, while not frustrating patients by over-challenging them with tasks they are not yet prepared to attempt.

Once agitation appears and treatment is deemed necessary, it is usually prudent to attempt nonpharmacological means to improve behavior if safety is not threatened and sufficient time is available to effect the desired change. Initial intervention is guided by identifying antecedents underlying the undesired behavior, then eliminating or modifying them to prevent its appearance. Agitation may arise from patient confusion, excessive environmental stimulation, uncomfortable medical conditions, and inappropriately challenging therapies. This realization can lead to fairly simple modifications in the patient's environment, changes in therapy location and/or composition, or treatment of specific medical problems that inhibit the appearance or easily and quickly ameliorate the presence of maladaptive behaviors. It is equally important for health care providers to recognize the differences between seemingly unusual behaviors that may in fact relate to particular cultural norms rather than to TBI-related behaviors.[30]

Behavioral modification is used when environmental alterations have not effected the desired change. This approach requires diligent identification of antecedent events, and a carefully coordinated and consistent interdisciplinary approach of the entire rehabilitation team and others involved in the day-to-day activities of the patient. An important aspect of behavior modification is an ongoing assessment of the plan's effectiveness with willingness to give it time to work and to change as needed. Effective strategies typically use a schedule of positive reinforcements without the application of negative reinforcements to enhance the emergence and long-term maintenance of adaptive behaviors.[30] The effectiveness of a plan is best determined by using a standardized assessment tool, such as the Overt Aggression Scale (OAS), both before and during the intervention. Behavioral modification plans are typically time consuming, but can be effective if all team members, including family members are educated regarding the rationale of the intervention and if enough time is provided to both assess the plan and change it as needed.

The first step in medication management is often to minimize or eliminate certain drugs that may potentially impair cognition and worsen behaviors, such as CNS depressants. However, when medication use is deemed necessary, adherence to some simple guidelines can be very helpful in achieving the desired results. A specific maladaptive behavior is targeted followed by the selection of an appropriate drug to modify it. Low dosages should be used initially with sufficient time given to effect a change. Objective behavior assessments, such as the OAS, can provide useful pre- and posttreatment data that help to determine treatment effectiveness. If agitation worsens one can change strategy, which may simply be to lower or eliminate the last medication change. It is also important to set a realistic target.[31] Doses should be titrated up slowly to monitor for side effects.

The most commonly used agents are mood stabilizers, antidepressants, novel antipsychotic medications, neurostimulants, β-blockers, and anxiolytic medications. Certain classes of medications such as benzodiazepines, anticholinergic agents, and traditional antipsychotics such as haloperidol that are used to treat agitation in other medical conditions are generally avoided as much as possible in the TBI population because of their sedating and cognitively impairing effects.[32,33]

Heterotopic Ossification

Heterotopic ossification (HO) is histologically normal-appearing bone in soft tissues. HO typically appears at the elbows, hips, shoulders, and knees following TBI, and can adversely affect range of motion and function. As HO progresses, it may entrap peripheral nerves resulting in neuropathies, and may ultimately cause complete joint ankylosis. Reported incidence of HO is highly variable, although is likely 10% to 20% following severe TBI.[34] Risk factors for developing HO increase with increasing injury severity and associated spasticity. Early clinical signs include joint pain with restricted range of motion, swelling, erythema, and increased warmth. Careful consideration must be given to rule out other causes of limb pain and swelling, including infection, venous thrombosis, complex regional pain syndrome, and undiagnosed trauma. Standard radiographs typically do not image HO until several weeks after clinical evidence becomes apparent. Therefore, radionuclide assessment is the preferred means for early detection. Early treatment options include diphosphonates and anti-inflammatory agents for up to 6 months. However, once medications are discontinued calcification of the bony matrix ensues, making this treatment controversial. Surgical resection is typically reserved for those who have restricted limb function but with evidence of well-preserved motor power, or for those who cannot be positioned adequately for care or other activities. Historically, resection was considered only after at least 18 months had passed and the bone appeared mature on radionuclide testing to limit the rate of recurrence. However, evidence suggests that earlier resection poses no additional reoccurrence risk as compared with late resection.[35]

Neuroendocrine Dysfunction

The location and tenuous vascular supply of the pituitary gland makes it vulnerable to injury in patients with TBI. Recent evidence has confirmed that moderate to severe TBI is frequently associated with pituitary abnormalities,[36–42] which can adversely impact rehabilitation outcomes,[43] body composition,[44] lipid profile,[44] mood, and quality of life.[45] In a recent review the Institute of Medicine reported, "there is sufficient evidence of an association between moderate or severe TBI and endocrine dysfunction, particularly hypopituitarism" and "sufficient evidence of an association between moderate or severe TBI and growth hormone insufficiency."[46] The onset of dysfunction is variable, appearing either shortly after TBI or up to 1 year later,[47] indicating the need to screen for neuroendocrine deficiencies at variable times after injury, including during inpatient rehabilitation.[48] Abnormalities may also be long lasting and accordingly require long-term treatment.[40]

Disorders of sodium metabolism are common following brain injury. Hypernatremia may be caused by dehydration, particularly when dysphagic patients are on modified diets that require them to ingest thickened fluids that are often taken in insufficient quantities. Less commonly, hypernatremia may be caused by diabetes insipidus during inpatient rehabilitation, which when present is associated with polydipsia and polyuria. Hyponatremia is among the most common metabolic alterations following TBI, although accurately determining its cause is difficult. The syndrome of inappropriate antidiuretic hormone secretion (SIADH) and cerebral salt wasting (CSW) both cause hyponatremia, but are differentiated based primarily on the fluid status of the patient. SIADH exists in patients with euvolumia and is managed by careful fluid restriction. CSW, however, is associated with hypovolumia and is treated with both sodium and fluid resuscitation. The markedly different treatment strategies make an accurate diagnosis critically important to prevent worsening clinical outcomes by exacerbating hypovolumia if CSW is misdiagnosed as SIADH. Other causes of hyponatremia should also be sought, including hypothyroidism, hypocortisolism, diuretic use, diarrhea, blood loss, emesis, and excessive sweating.

Spasticity

Spasticity, defined as a velocity-dependent increase in passive stretch of a joint, is a common post-TBI problem that adversely impacts joint range of motion, ADL performance, and mobility. When present, it often consumes a disproportionate time of the rehabilitation process and increases the burden on care providers. Spasticity therefore requires immediate treatment when identified to prevent joint contractures and restrictions in mobility as well as ADL performance. Initial treatment typically includes aggressive stretching by all members of the rehabilitation team, including family members and patients when feasible. This stretching is accompanied by various modalities, such as application of heat and cold that serve to increase joint flexibility and decrease spasticity. Braces are often applied to provide sustained stretching of spastic muscles. Carefully applied plaster casts may also be used across a spastic elbow, knee, or ankle, which permits sustained stretch over a period of days to weeks, resulting in more effective and efficient improvement in range of motion.

Enteral medications including baclofen, tizanidine, benzodiazepines, and dantrolene can be used to decrease spasticity, although sedating and cognitively impairing effects often limit their usefulness in patients with TBI. Selective motor point blocks with phenol or purified botulinum toxin effectively reduces spasticity at the site of injections, noting that treatments typically need to be repeated every few months. Intrathecally administered baclofen is an alternative means to decrease spasticity. This approach concentrates baclofen close to its theorized site of action in the spinal cord, significantly improving spasticity control while limiting undesirable cerebral effects of fatigue and impaired cognition. It also permits more controlled relief of spasticity as certain patients may require some degree of spasticity to improve transfer and ambulation performance. Prolonged spasticity may result in joint contractures that are not responsive to previously mentioned management strategies. Surgical interventions such as tendon lengthening and tenotomies may become necessary to improve patient positioning, hygiene, and overall functional skills.

Disorders of Consciousness

Disorders of consciousness (DOC) including coma, the vegetative state, and minimally conscious state are among the most challenging conditions for rehabilitation providers and the most frustrating for families and loved ones. Widespread loss of neuronal connectivity following TBI is believed to underlie the clinical condition of DOC, accounting for these patients' altered awareness of self and environment. Confusion exists regarding the various terms describing DOC as well as how best to accurately ascertain the correct diagnosis. Coma is a state of unconsciousness marked by nonarousal to stimulation and the lack of sleep-wake cycles. Coma is a self-limited condition, lasting 2 to 4 weeks, followed by either death or emergence into another state of consciousness. The vegetative state is a condition of presumed unawareness manifested by the apparent inability to purposefully interact with self or environments but with the reemergence of sleep-wake cycles and intermittent eye opening. In the minimally conscious state there is intermittent but definite evidence of self or environmental awareness.[49] No definitive treatments exist to improve arousal or emergence from DOC, although several have been proposed, with some evidence supporting their utility. Administration of dopaminergic drugs such as levadopa[50–53] and amantadine[54,55] have been reported to be beneficial, although both require further study to better ascertain their effectiveness. Zolpidem has also been reported to paradoxically improve arousal,[56] although it appears that very few individuals have a favorable response and inadequate data exist to predict who will respond.[57] Other interventions have been proposed, including median nerve stimulation,[58,59] extradural cortical electrical stimulation,[60] and intrathecal baclofen,[53] although insufficient evidence is available to provide treatment guidelines. Deep brain stimulation of the central thalamus has been reported to induce favorable behavioral changes in a man in the minimally conscious state of 6 years' duration.[61] Regardless of methods used to enhance awareness, it is imperative to maintain skin integrity, pulmonary hygiene, and joint flexibility in patients with DOC following TBI.

Seizures

Post-traumatic seizures are categorized depending on the timing of their occurrence. Immediate seizures occur within 24 hours of trauma; early seizures within the first week, and late seizures after the first week post trauma. Seizures are common post-TBI sequelae, with a standardized incidence of 17% after severe TBI.[62] However, other factors increase the risk, including the presence of multiple contusions, subdural hemorrhages, depressed skull fractures, older age, early seizures, multiple cranial operations, and large midline shift.[62,63] Adequate management of posttraumatic seizures is critical, as they have been associated with premature mortality after TBI.[64–68] However, routine prophylaxis for late seizures in all individuals with TBI is not recommended because no study has yet found that it effectively reduces its frequency,[69–72] and certain anticonvulsants can worsen cognitive skills.[73,74] In general, patients with TBI admitted for rehabilitation who have not had a seizure are taken off of anticonvulsants unless they have other risk factors that may warrant continued use. When anticonvulsants are deemed necessary, most rehabilitation specialists tend to choose the newer agents, which are generally thought to have a less notable impact on cognitive performance.[75]

Hydrocephalus

Posttraumatic symptomatic hydrocephalus is a well-recognized condition, although its true incidence is uncertain and is widely reported as 0.7%[76] to 29%[77] because of varying criteria used to make the diagnosis. Posttraumatic hydrocephalus should be suspected clinically when there is a decline in a patient's neurological, cognitive, or behavioral condition or when clinical improvement unexpectedly ceases during the rehabilitation process. Diagnosis is typically made by the presence of the clinical signs described, in addition to neuroimaging that reveals enlarged ventricles out of proportion to the sulci and periventricular edema. High-volume drainage of cerebrospinal fluid (CSF) may be useful to aid the diagnostic process, with temporary improvement in clinical performance indicating the presence of hydrocephalus and the likelihood of successful intervention. Treatment is CSF shunting, which can significantly improve rehabilitation outcomes in properly selected patients.

SUMMARY

Neurorehabilitation is a growing field that is constantly innovating on all fronts. As we learn more about the brain's capability for recovery, new rehabilitation theories emerge that ignite further research, which will lead to the development of new therapeutic interventions. What will likely remain constant is the need for an interdisciplinary approach to TBI rehabilitation that takes advantage of the skills of each individual discipline while combining the strengths of all team members to effectively address common problems that affect multiple domains of function. Given the multitude of medical, cognitive, and behavioral problems associated with TBI, diligent attention to each individual is critical in maximizing outcomes and enhancing the possibility of community reintegration.

REFERENCES

1. Granger CV, Markello SJ, Graham JE, et al. The uniform data system for medical rehabilitation: report of patients with traumatic brain injury discharged from rehabilitation programs in 2000-2007. Am J Phys Med Rehabil 2010;89(4):265–78.
2. Hoffman JM, Doctor JN, Chan L, et al. Potential impact of the new Medicare prospective payment system on reimbursement for traumatic brain injury inpatient rehabilitation. Arch Phys Med Rehabil 2003;84(8):1165–72.
3. Born J, Wagner U. Awareness in memory: being explicit about the role of sleep. Trends Cogn Sci 2004;8(6):242–4.
4. Walker MP. A refined model of sleep and the time course of memory formation. Behav Brain Sci 2005;28(1):51–64 [discussion: 64–104].
5. Shadmehr R, Holcomb HH. Neural correlates of motor memory consolidation. Science 1997;277(5327):821–5.
6. Stolze H, Klebe S, Zechlin C, et al. Falls in frequent neurological diseases—prevalence, risk factors and aetiology. J Neurol 2004;251(1):79–84.
7. Collicut MJ. Fear of falling after brain injury. Clin Rehabil 2008;22:635–45.
8. Teasell R, McRae M, Foley N, et al. The incidence and consequences of falls in stroke patients during inpatient rehabilitation: factors associated with high risk. Arch Phys Med Rehabil 2002;83(3):329–33.
9. Ziino C, Ponsford J. Selective attention deficits and subjective fatigue following traumatic brain injury. Neuropsychology 2006;20(3):383–90.
10. Ouellet MC, Beaulieu-Bonneau S, Morin CM. Insomnia in patients with traumatic brain injury: frequency, characteristics, and risk factors. J Head Trauma Rehabil 2006;21(3):199–212.
11. Kreutzer JS, Seel RT, Gourley E. The prevalence and symptom rates of depression after traumatic brain injury: a comprehensive examination. Brain Inj 2001; 15(7):563–76.
12. Castriotta RJ, Wilde MC, Lai JM, et al. Prevalence and consequences of sleep disorders in traumatic brain injury. J Clin Sleep Med 2007;3(4):349–56.
13. Rao V, Spiro J, Vaishnavi S, et al. Prevalence and types of sleep disturbances acutely after traumatic brain injury. Brain Inj 2008;22(5):381–6.
14. Cohen M, Oksenberg A, Snir D, et al. Temporally related changes of sleep complaints in traumatic brain injured patients. J Neurol Neurosurg Psychiatry 1992;55(4):313–5.
15. Harada M, Minami R, Hattori E, et al. Sleep in brain-damaged patients. An all night sleep study of 105 cases. Kumamoto Med J 1976;29(3):110–27.
16. Zeitzer JM, Friedman L, O'Hara R. Insomnia in the context of traumatic brain injury. J Rehabil Res Dev 2009;46(6):827–36.
17. Mendelson WB. A review of the evidence for the efficacy and safety of trazodone in insomnia. J Clin Psychiatry 2005;66(4):469–76.
18. Zammit G. Comparative tolerability of newer agents for insomnia. Drug Saf 2009; 32(9):735–48.
19. Blackman JA, Patrick PD, Buck ML, et al. Paroxysmal autonomic instability with dystonia after brain injury. Arch Neurol 2004;61(3):321–8.
20. Boeve BF, Wijdicks EF, Benarroch EE, et al. Paroxysmal sympathetic storms ("diencephalic seizures") after severe diffuse axonal head injury. Mayo Clin Proc 1998;73(2):148–52.

21. Baguley IJ, Cameron ID, Green AM, et al. Pharmacological management of dysautonomia following traumatic brain injury. Brain Inj 2004;18(5):409–17.

22. Rossitch E Jr, Bullard DE. The autonomic dysfunction syndrome: aetiology and treatment. Br J Neurosurg 1988;2(4):471–8.

23. Wang VY, Manley G. Recognition of paroxysmal autonomic instability with dystonia (PAID) in a patient with traumatic brain injury. J Trauma 2008;64(2):500–2.

24. Rabinstein AA, Benarroch EE. Treatment of paroxysmal sympathetic hyperactivity. Curr Treat Options Neurol 2008;10(2):151–7.

25. Kim Y, Kim K. Effects of single-dose methylphenidate on cognitive performance in patients with traumatic brain injury: a double-blind placebo-controlled study. Clin Rehabil 2006;20:24–30.

26. Whyte J, Vaccaro M, Grieb-Neff P, et al. The effects of bromocriptine on attention deficits after traumatic brain injury: a placebo-controlled pilot study. Am J Phys Med Rehabil 2008;87(2):85–99.

27. Neurobehavioral Guidelines Working Group, Warden DL, Gordon B, et al. Guidelines for the pharmacologic treatment of neurobehavioral sequelae of traumatic brain injury. J Neurotrauma 2006;23(10):1468–501.

28. Silver JM, Koumaras B, Chen M, et al. Effects of rivastigmine on cognitive function in patients with traumatic brain injury. Neurology 2006;67(5):748–55.

29. Sandel ME, Mysiw WJ. The agitated brain injured patient. Part 1: definitions, differential diagnosis, and assessment. Arch Phys Med Rehabil 1996;77(6):617–23.

30. Karol RL. Principles of behavioral analysis and modification. In: Zasler ND, Katz DI, Zafonte RD, editors. Brain injury medicine: principles and practice. 1st edition. New York: Demos; 2007. p. 815–33.

31. Silver JM, Arciniegas DB. Pharmacotherapy of neuropsychiatric disturbances. In: Zasler ND, Katz DI, Zafonte RD, editors. Brain injury medicine: principles and practice. 1st edition. New York: Demos; 2007. p. 963–93.

32. Levy M, Berson A, Cook T, et al. Treatment of agitation following traumatic brain injury: a review of the literature. NeuroRehabilitation 2005;20(4):279–306.

33. Mysiw WJ, Bogner JA, Corrigan JD, et al. The impact of acute care medications on rehabilitation outcome after traumatic brain injury. Brain Inj 2006;20(9):905–11.

34. Garland DE. Surgical approaches for resection of heterotopic ossification in traumatic brain-injured adults. Clin Orthop Relat Res 1991;(263):59–70.

35. Chalidis B, Stengel D, Giannoudis PV. Early excision and late excision of heterotopic ossification after traumatic brain injury are equivalent: a systematic review of the literature. J Neurotrauma 2007;24(11):1675–86.

36. Kelly DF, Gonzalo IT, Cohan P, et al. Hypopituitarism following traumatic brain injury and aneurysmal subarachnoid hemorrhage: a preliminary report. J Neurosurg 2000;93(5):743–52.

37. Lieberman SA, Oberoi AL, Gilkison CR, et al. Prevalence of neuroendocrine dysfunction in patients recovering from traumatic brain injury. J Clin Endocrinol Metab 2001;86(6):2752–6.

38. Agha A, Thornton E, O'Kelly P, et al. Posterior pituitary dysfunction after traumatic brain injury. J Clin Endocrinol Metab 2004;89(12):5987–92.

39. Aimaretti G, Ambrosio MR, Di Somma C, et al. Hypopituitarism induced by traumatic brain injury in the transition phase. J Endocrinol Invest 2005;28(11):984–9.

40. Bondanelli M, De Marinis L, Ambrosio MR, et al. Occurrence of pituitary dysfunction following traumatic brain injury. J Neurotrauma 2004;21(6):685–96.

41. Leal-Cerro A, Flores JM, Rincon M, et al. Prevalence of hypopituitarism and growth hormone deficiency in adults long-term after severe traumatic brain injury. Clin Endocrinol (Oxf) 2005;62(5):525–32.

42. Schneider HJ, Schneider M, Saller B, et al. Prevalence of anterior pituitary insufficiency 3 and 12 months after traumatic brain injury. Eur J Endocrinol 2006; 154(2):259–65.

43. Bondanelli M, Ambrosio MR, Cavazzini L, et al. Anterior pituitary function may predict functional and cognitive outcome in patients with traumatic brain injury undergoing rehabilitation. J Neurotrauma 2007;24(11):1687–97.

44. Klose M, Watt T, Brennum J, et al. Posttraumatic hypopituitarism is associated with an unfavorable body composition and lipid profile, and decreased quality of life 12 months after injury. J Clin Endocrinol Metab 2007;92(10): 3861–8.

45. Kelly DF, McArthur DL, Levin H, et al. Neurobehavioral and quality of life changes associated with growth hormone insufficiency after complicated mild, moderate, or severe traumatic brain injury. J Neurotrauma 2006;23(6):928–42.

46. Gulf war and health. In: Long-term consequences of traumatic brain injury, vol. 7. Washington, DC: The National Academies; 2009. Available at: http://books.nap. edu/openbook.php?record_id=12436. Accessed September 1, 2010.

47. Giordano G, Aimaretti G, Ghigo E. Variations of pituitary function over time after brain injuries: the lesson from a prospective study. Pituitary 2005;8(3–4):227–31.

48. Ghigo E, Masel B, Aimaretti G, et al. Consensus guidelines on screening for hypopituitarism following traumatic brain injury. Brain Inj 2005;19(9):711–24.

49. Giacino JT, Ashwal S, Childs N, et al. The minimally conscious state: definition and diagnostic criteria. Neurology 2002;58(3):349–53.

50. Matsuda W, Matsumura A, Komatsu Y, et al. Awakenings from persistent vegetative state: report of three cases with parkinsonism and brain stem lesions on MRI. J Neurol Neurosurg Psychiatry 2003;74(11):1571–3.

51. Haig AJ, Ruess JM. Recovery from vegetative state of six months' duration associated with Sinemet (levodopa/carbidopa). Arch Phys Med Rehabil 1990;71(13): 1081–3.

52. Koeda T, Takeshita K. A case report of remarkable improvement of motor disturbances with L-dopa in a patient with post-diffuse axonal injury. Brain Dev 1998; 20(2):124–6.

53. Sara M, Pistoia F, Mura E, et al. Intrathecal baclofen in patients with persistent vegetative state: 2 hypotheses. Arch Phys Med Rehabil 2009;90(7):1245–9.

54. Zafonte RD, Watanabe T, Mann NR. Amantadine: a potential treatment for the minimally conscious state. Brain Inj 1998;12(7):617–21.

55. Whyte J, Katz D, Long D, et al. Predictors of outcome in prolonged posttraumatic disorders of consciousness and assessment of medication effects: a multicenter study. Arch Phys Med Rehabil 2005;86(3):453–62.

56. Clauss R, Nel W. Drug induced arousal from the permanent vegetative state. NeuroRehabilitation 2006;21(1):23–8.

57. Whyte J, Myers R. Incidence of clinically significant responses to zolpidem among patients with disorders of consciousness: a preliminary placebo controlled trial. Am J Phys Med Rehabil 2009;88(5):410–8.

58. Liu JT, Wang CH, Chou IC, et al. Regaining consciousness for prolonged comatose patients with right median nerve stimulation. Acta Neurochir Suppl 2003;87: 11–4.

59. Cooper EB, Cooper JB. Electrical treatment of coma via the median nerve. Acta Neurochir Suppl 2003;87:7–10.

60. Canavero S, Massa-Micon B, Cauda F, et al. Bifocal extradural cortical stimulation-induced recovery of consciousness in the permanent post-traumatic vegetative state. J Neurol 2009;256(5):834–6.

61. Schiff ND, Giacino JT, Kalmar K, et al. Behavioural improvements with thalamic stimulation after severe traumatic brain injury. Nature 2007;448(7153):600–3.

62. Annegers JF, Hauser WA, Coan SP, et al. A population-based study of seizures after traumatic brain injuries. N Engl J Med 1998;338(1):20–4.

63. Englander J, Bushnik T, Duong TT, et al. Analyzing risk factors for late posttraumatic seizures: a prospective, multicenter investigation. Arch Phys Med Rehabil 2003;84(3):365–73.

64. Harrison-Felix C, Whiteneck G, DeVivo M, et al. Mortality following rehabilitation in the traumatic brain injury model systems of care. NeuroRehabilitation 2004;19(1): 45–54.

65. Corkin S, Sullivan EV, Carr FA. Prognostic factors for life expectancy after penetrating head injury. Arch Neurol 1984;41(9):975–7.

66. Weiss GH, Caveness WF, Einsiedel-Lechtape H, et al. Life expectancy and causes of death in a group of head-injured veterans of World War I. Arch Neurol 1982;39(12):741–3.

67. Walker AE, Leuchs HK, Lechtape-Gruter H, et al. Life expectancy of head injured men with and without epilepsy. Arch Neurol 1971;24(2):95–100.

68. Shavelle RM, Strauss D, Whyte J, et al. Long-term causes of death after traumatic brain injury. Am J Phys Med Rehabil 2001;80(7):510–6 [quiz: 517–9].

69. Temkin NR. Antiepileptogenesis and seizure prevention trials with antiepileptic drugs: meta-analysis of controlled trials. Epilepsia 2001;42(4):515–24.

70. Temkin NR, Dikmen SS, Wilensky AJ, et al. A randomized, double-blind study of phenytoin for the prevention of post-traumatic seizures. N Engl J Med 1990; 323(8):497–502.

71. Temkin NR. Preventing and treating posttraumatic seizures: the human experience. Epilepsia 2009;50(Suppl 2):10–3.

72. Teasell R, Bayona N, Lippert C, et al. Post-traumatic seizure disorder following acquired brain injury. Brain Inj 2007;21(2):201–14.

73. Dikmen SS, Temkin NR, Miller B, et al. Neurobehavioral effects of phenytoin prophylaxis of posttraumatic seizures. JAMA 1991;265(10):1271–7.

74. Meador KJ, Loring DW, Abney OL, et al. Effects of carbamazepine and phenytoin on EEG and memory in healthy adults. Epilepsia 1993;34(1):153–7.

75. Crooks CY, Zumsteg JM, Bell KR. Traumatic brain injury: a review of practice management and recent advances. Phys Med Rehabil Clin N Am 2007;18(4): 681–710.

76. Cardoso ER, Galbraith S. Posttraumatic hydrocephalus—a retrospective review. Surg Neurol 1985;23(3):261–4.

77. Hawkins TD, Lloyd AD, Fletcher GI, et al. Ventricular size following head injury: a clinicoradiological study. Clin Radiol 1976;27(3):279–89.

Role and Impact of Cognitive Rehabilitation

Kristen Dams-O'Connor, PhD*, Wayne A. Gordon, PhD

KEYWORDS

• Cognitive rehabilitation • Cognitive impairment • Brain injury

Individuals with traumatic brain injury (TBI) often experience impairments in cognitive, behavioral, physical, and emotional functioning that impact their ability to work productively, maintain social relationships, participate in the community, and function independently.[1] All people with a TBI are unique in terms of the constellation of consequences they experience, the personal meaning of their losses, and the impact of these losses on their own life. Most individuals who sustain severe-to-moderate injuries, and many of those with milder injuries, experience a range of enduring challenges.[2–5] In the cognitive arena, brain injury results in prototypical deficits in attention, processing speed, memory, and executive functioning.[6,7] In addition, alterations to neuromodulatory systems affect cognition, mood, and behavior.[8,9] Behavioral and emotional consequences of TBI may include depression, anxiety, post-traumatic stress disorder, impulsivity, and agitation/aggression.[1,10,11] Physical symptoms include fatigue, headaches, balance problems, seizures, and endocrine dysfunction.[12] Although the severity of these impairments is often ameliorated over time and with rehabilitation, for some individuals these impairments become chronic and can be associated with high rates of unemployment, mood disorders, anxiety disorders, substance abuse, incarceration, and homelessness.[13,14]

Cognitive rehabilitation refers to various theoretically based and empirically validated interventions that have been designed to maximize cognitive functioning and thereby minimize the functional consequences of post-TBI cognitive and behavioral impairments. Broadly speaking, cognitive rehabilitation teaches individuals the cognitive skills necessary to perform tasks that they were able to do before their injury but not able to do following their injury. Treatment may focus on improving function in any

This work was supported by Grant Number H133B040033, National Institute on Disability and Rehabilitation Research, US Department of Education; Grant Number 5R49-CE-001171, Centers for Disease Control and Prevention.
Department of Rehabilitation Medicine, Mount Sinai School of Medicine, One Gustave L. Levy Place, Box 1240, New York, NY 10029-6574, USA
* Corresponding author.
E-mail address: Kristen.dams-o'connor@mountsinai.org

or all of the following domains: attention, visual perception, memory, learning, and executive functioning (ie, organization, planning, or problem solving). Emotional regulation, mood, social skills training, and community integration also may be targets of interventions. Sessions may be rendered in individual or group settings, or (more recently) via supervised computer or telephone sessions. While individual treatment goals vary depending on the severity of injury, the person's premorbid academic or vocational achievement and the nature and severity of the person's cognitive, behavioral, physical, and emotional difficulties, the overall goal of cognitive rehabilitation is to assist the individual to improve their day-to-day functioning to the greatest extent possible given his or her limitations.[15]

MEASURING THE IMPACT OF COGNITIVE REHABILITATION

Although much more research is needed, a large body of evidence exists supporting the effectiveness of cognitive rehabilitation in individuals with TBI.[16–20] Even more anecdotal evidence exists describing the ways in which individuals who successfully complete cognitive rehabilitation programs go on to live more productive, fulfilling lives as contributing members of their families and communities. It is unfortunate that these gains are not always reflected in statistically significant changes in the outcome measures used in a given study.

There are many factors that make it difficult to measure the impact of cognitive interventions. One major barrier is the poor ecological validity of neuropsychological tests, which makes it difficult to demonstrate the impact of cognitive rehabilitation on real-world outcomes (ie, productivity, community integration, or quality of interpersonal relationships). For example, the relationship between a psychometric measure of sustained attention and the ability to follow a dinner table conversation has not been demonstrated. Research is able to quantify proximal changes in discrete cognitive abilities to measure treatment outcome, but there is a dearth of outcome measures that adequately operationalize and quantify real-world outcomes.[17] Another barrier to establishing the efficacy of interventions for individuals with TBI is the heterogeneity of etiology, severity, symptom presentation, and the diversity of ways the various cognitive and behavioral impairments impact day-to-day function.[21] To date the differential characteristics of those who do and do not benefit from treatment have not been identified. Finally, it is often difficult to follow participants for long periods of time following the cessation of treatment, so information on continued progress or decline in function is not available.[22]

Roles of Cognitive Rehabilitation

Cognitive rehabilitation plays many roles in the process of recovery. The cognitive, behavioral, and emotional sequelae of TBI often interact and create havoc in terms of their impact on an individual's day-to-day functioning and quality of life. Thus cognitive rehabilitation interventions are often designed to target multiple aspects of function. In fact, it is relatively uncommon for interventions to focus exclusively on one functional domain without directly or indirectly addressing difficulties in other domains. The many roles that cognitive rehabilitation can have in impacting the lives of individuals with TBI are described.

Role 1: restoration of function

A distinction has been made in the literature between the two general approaches to cognitive rehabilitation: restoration or recovery of lost function and compensation. Restorative interventions are designed to restore the neural circuitry underlying impaired cognitive processes by using practice and focused training exercises to promote their systematic engagement. These interventions are based on the notion that neuroplasticity provides an opportunity to support the re-establishment of damaged neural circuits.[23] Restoration of function is often a primary goal of individuals with TBI, as quite understandably they hope to return to preinjury levels of functioning.

There is growing evidence that basic cognitive abilities, such as reaction time and attention, can be directly restored through exercises designed to stimulate the neurological circuitry supporting these functions.[17,24] For example, some evidence suggests that directly training the working memory system with repetitive practice can result in improvements in attention and self-reported improvements in everyday functioning.[25] Similarly, a specialized computer training program that targets working memory skills resulted in improvements in working memory and attention and self-reported cognitive functioning among stroke patients.[26] Another example of the this type of intervention is the use of constraint-induced movement therapy (CMIT) to restore language skills. CMIT is a treatment that involves the application of systematic massed practice of verbal responses to restore language skills that have become impaired by the injury and subsequent learned nonuse. It has been demonstrated that language skills in individuals with chronic aphasia secondary to left hemisphere stroke can be improved by reversing their learned nonuse.[27,28] In other words, the communication skills of aphasics can be improved by creating situations in which they are forced to speak.

Pilot research recently conducted at the Brain Injury Research Center (BIRC) at Mount Sinai School of Medicine (MSSM) explored the usability of a neuroplasticity-based computerized cognitive training program in a sample of 10 community-dwelling individuals with TBI 6 months to 22 years after injury. The program is designed to facilitate neurological restoration of impaired circuitry underlying specific cognitive processes by directly engaging and challenging foundational cognitive skills.[29,30] Participants used the software at home for up to 40 minutes per day, 5 days per week for 6 weeks. Following treatment, improvements were noted on one or more standardized neuropsychological assessment measures for all participants, and all patients reported fewer everyday cognitive failures after testing.[31]

In general, although there is some evidence that direct restorative training has beneficial effects on trained functions, the evidence is not sufficient to support the impact of restorative training alone (ie, without additional training in compensatory or metacognitive strategies).[17]

Many cognitive interventions incorporate both direct restorative interventions and compensatory strategy training to maximize treatment results and to enhance generalization of learned skills to community activities. For example, the impact of constraint-induced language therapies on functional communication is maximized when additional compensatory training in everyday communication is provided.[28] Another example of this integrative approach is the finding that direct attention training using sequential exercises that aim to restore the attentional system can be effective when applied within metacognitive strategy training.[32,33] Similarly, visual restoration training has been found to have a significant impact on visual spatial skills when it is combined with compensatory cueing.[34]

Role 2: compensatory strategy training

The most common role of cognitive rehabilitation involves assisting an individual to compensate for impaired abilities through the use of learned internal or external strategies. These strategies are essentially substitutes for lost abilities and are designed to minimize the functional impact of injury-related impairments.[35] Training in the use of compensatory strategies requires an individualized assessment of a person's cognitive strengths and weaknesses to identify both impaired functions and intact abilities. This allows a clinician and client to develop individualized strategies that can be supported by intact abilities, thereby circumventing the impaired cognitive functions. Compensation also may involve learning general rules or heuristics that provide step-by-step procedures to help a person to solve problems, regulate his or her behaviors, or perform daily activities. While the implementation of compensatory strategies may become more habitual and even automatic over time and with continued use, continuous lifelong implementation of these learned strategies is required if day-to-day function outcomes are to be achieved.[35]

Attention Impairments in concentration and information processing are characteristic sequelae of TBI. Evidence indicates that cognitive rehabilitation aimed at teaching time pressure management (TPM) strategies ameliorates functional impairments related to slowed information processing and complex attention.[36] TPM interventions are designed to teach the person to compensate for reduced processing speed by learning to allow sufficient time to manage particular tasks through the use of strategies (eg, asking for information to be repeated, clarifying information, and anticipating task demands). Attention process training (APT) is another intervention that has a large evidence base demonstrating the impact of this theory-driven systematic approach to attention training.[37] APT tasks are organized hierarchically to exercise components of attention, beginning with sustained attention skills and working up to selective, alternating, and divided attention. Throughout training, strategies to maximize performance are practiced in session, and homework is used to maximize generalization of learned skills. In general, interventions that emphasize the development of compensatory strategies (such as removing environmental distractions, taking breaks, and using cues to remain attentive) have a significant impact on complex attention functions such as attention regulation and information processing.[17]

Memory There is considerable evidence to support the impact of compensatory strategy training on improving memory function among individuals with TBI independent of severity and time since injury.[17] Some of the approaches that have a significant impact include visual imagery training[38] and training in the use of external aids such as a memory diary (Ownsworth and McFarland, 1999)[39] or a portable pager (Wilson and colleagues, 2001, 2005).[40,41] When external memory aids are taught in combination with self-instructional strategies, the functional impact of external tools is enhanced.[39] An errorless learning approach to strategy training can help even severely injured individuals learn specific behaviors or procedures, such as writing emails or other personally relevant tasks.[42–44] Errorless learning involves providing sufficient cues during training so that an individual can only provide a correct response. Over time cues are sequentially reduced so that an individual is able to perform the desired task error-free with minimal cueing. This approach can help prevent individuals with severe memory impairment from remembering incorrect responses or mistakes instead of accurate information.

Executive functions Metacognitive strategy training has consistently been shown to improve daily problem-solving abilities.[20] For example, training in the use of metacognitive approaches to problem-solving that incorporate emotional self-regulation strategies designed to facilitate clear thinking has been shown to improve general executive functioning and problem-solving behavior.[45] In addition, external cueing of autobiographical memories relevant to the task at hand (ie, cueing recollection of the last time a particular task was successfully performed) has been shown to help people to plan everyday tasks.[46] Goal management training (GMT) is another compensatory strategy that has been found to have a positive impact on daily activities.[47] GMT involves training individuals to stop and think about what they are doing, identify a specific goal, delineate the steps or subordinate goals that must be completed to meet this goal, and then review the outcome to verify that the selected goal has been achieved.[47] In general, metacognitive training to learn problem-solving strategies, self-regulation training, and systematic application of learned strategies to everyday activities can have a considerable impact on the functioning of individuals with TBI.[17]

Role 3: increase awareness

It is not surprising that unawareness of cognitive, behavioral, and emotional impairments is common among individuals with TBI, as the organ that coordinates self-observation and appraisal is altered by the injury. Even when individuals can name or describe their injury-related impairments, they may not recognize the consequences these impairments may have on their day-to-day functioning. This results in unrealistic goal setting, unsafe choices, refusal to learn or use compensatory strategies, and multiple failures. Unawareness is commonly recognized as a significant barrier to treatment.[48] Accordingly, an important role of cognitive rehabilitation is helping an individual to become aware of injury-related deficits and their functional implications.

Interventions specifically designed to increase awareness of deficits have been shown to have a significant impact on self-appraisal, appropriate goal setting, and error monitoring. These interventions provide education about TBI and individualized feedback on performance. For example, participants may do exercises in which they predict their performance on particular tasks and then monitor and evaluate the outcomes as a means of increasing awareness of any discrepancy between expectations and true abilities.[49,50] Additional strategies such as using verbal self-regulation during performance of personally relevant tasks and actively anticipating potential pitfalls before initiating a task can further enhance the impact of awareness-raising interventions.[49,51]

Given the potential negative impact of deficit unawareness in fostering motivation, engagement, and involvement in treatment, raising awareness is often recognized as a necessary prerequisite for successful rehabilitation,[48] and accordingly awareness interventions are frequently embedded in cognitive interventions. This might involve asking patients to predict how they think they might perform on specific tasks, monitor performance, evaluate their own performance, and identify factors contributing to failures and successes. Holistic cognitive rehabilitation programs commonly incorporate group interventions in which participants give and receive performance-related feedback, in addition to individual psychotherapy to help individuals deal with personal losses.

Role 4: improve mood and regulate emotions

Major depressive disorder (MDD) has been shown to occur in 25% to 61% of individuals with TBI.[10,52,53] High rates of depression are unrelated to severity of TBI or time since injury.[54] Research documents alarmingly high rates of suicidal ideation (21% to 22%) and suicide attempts (18%) among individuals with TBI,[55] which far exceed rates found in individuals without TBI.[56] Due to the various cognitive, physical, and emotional changes after a TBI, individuals with TBI are constantly confronted with things they cannot do as well as or the same way they did before the accident. Each time this happens, they are confronted with the discrepancy between previous and current abilities, which can cause overwhelming feelings of loss and trigger frustration, depression, and anxiety. Depression can also directly result from damage to neurological circuitry in the frontal, temporal, limbic, and basal ganglia regions of the brain.[57,58] In addition, depression and anxiety can exacerbate cognitive deficits,[54] thereby compounding the functional impairments experienced by many individuals with TBI.

There is growing evidence that interventions based on cognitive behavioral treatment (CBT) approaches can be effective in the treatment of depression and other mood symptoms among individuals with TBI.[54] CBT refers to psychotherapeutic interventions that aim to help an individual to recognize how thoughts influence feelings and behaviors, and use this awareness to gain control over mood, emotional reactions, and behaviors.[59] CBT interventions commonly incorporate in vivo practice of strategies, homework to enhance carryover and relevance of learned strategies, and keeping records of emotional triggers, feelings, thoughts, and behaviors. These characteristics make CBT easily modifiable for use with individuals with cognitive impairments, given the inherent structure, repetition, and record keeping involved in the interventions.[60] For example, a cognitive behavioral anger management program has been shown to successfully help participants to become aware of their cognitive, physical, and emotional reactions to environmental stimuli, and use self-instructional strategies to manage anger.[61] Moreover, emotional regulation appears to be an important mitigating factor in the impact of cognitive rehabilitation, and cognitive interventions that include training in emotional control tend to have a strong impact on functional outcomes.[45]

Role 5: return to work

Given that a large proportion of TBI survivors are injured during young adulthood, the ability to return to and maintain gainful employment is a common rehabilitation goal. Unemployment rates among individuals with TBI are reported to be well over 70%,[62,63] and it is widely recognized that cognitive, behavioral, and personality impairments present greater barriers to employment than do physical ones.[64] Documented unemployment rates do not adequately reflect underemployment, which can be associated with a loss of prestige and identity, and can be a major determinant of satisfaction and quality of life.

Although the type, duration, and intensity of interventions included in meta-analytic reviews examining the effectiveness of cognitive rehabilitation in enhancing vocational outcomes vary, the evidence generally indicates that individuals who receive cognitive interventions are more likely to return to work than those who do not receive treatment.[65,66] Many factors in addition to cognitive impairments interact to create barriers to gainful employment, such as emotional dysregulation, low awareness of deficits, fatigue, and impulsive behaviors.[64,66] Accordingly, the factors influencing an individual's employability are commonly addressed in the context of comprehensive or holistic cognitive rehabilitation programs that are designed to address multiple areas of functioning. Indeed, many comprehensive programs identify returning to work as a distal treatment goal, and measure long-term success of the intervention in terms of post-treatment employment rates. Across studies on comprehensive or holistic cognitive rehabilitation programs, between 39% and 62% of participants engage in community-based employment after completing treatment.[17]

Role 6: community integration

The ability to interact and communicate effectively with others is an essential component of social integration and participation in the community. Social and communication deficits such as impulsiveness, egocentricity, inappropriate responding, and reduced initiation can, over time, lead to isolation and reduced quality of life. Cognitive rehabilitation can play an important role in helping individuals to learn social pragmatics, communication skills, and social behaviors that support reintegration into the community. There is ample evidence that cognitive rehabilitation programs that teach pragmatic communication skills, social behaviors, and social perception skills[67,68] improve functional communication. Successful approaches tend to incorporate training in specific behaviors (greetings, topic selection), social perception (interpreting facial expressions), self-monitoring, and individual goal setting.[67,68] Involving family members in treatment can enhance carryover of learned skills to community settings.[69] In general, rehabilitation interventions that focus on social communication and metacognitive strategy training have a significant impact on functional communication skills, social adaptiveness, psychosocial functioning (participation/integration), and quality of life.[20,69,68]

Given the breadth of skills and factors that contribute to successful community integration after TBI, it is not surprising that comprehensive or holistic neuropsychological rehabilitation programs that integrate cognitive and interpersonal interventions have a considerable impact on this domain. Holistic programs tend to incorporate individual and group therapies that emphasize metacognitive compensatory strategies, regulation of emotions, interpersonal skills training, and functional adaptive skill training.[69] Holistic rehabilitation has been shown to have a greater impact on community functioning and overall productivity than traditional multidisciplinary (occupational therapy, physical therapy, and speech therapy) postacute rehabilitation programs.[70] Several studies indicate that comprehensive holistic rehabilitation interventions have a significant impact on community functioning, social participation, productivity, and quality of life.[17]

Role 7: prevention of self-injurious and antisocial behavior

Individuals with TBI are at high risk for alcohol and substance abuse[13,71] due to disruptions in impulse control, poor self-regulation, and a need to self-medicate injury-related cognitive, behavioral, or emotional symptoms that are not adequately treated. Although substance use predates an injury for some individuals, many turn to substances in an effort to cope with the devastating losses resulting from their injury. In addition to the health consequences associated with substance use in the general population, alcohol and drug use can exacerbate injury-related cognitive impairments in individuals with TBI, intensifying language problems, poor balance, impulsivity, and aggressiveness.[72] Substance use also can cause dangerous drug interactions with prescription medications.[72] Finally, substance use may be implicated in the development of other negative outcomes, such as homelessness and incarceration.[73,74] Taken together, it is not surprising that individuals with TBI are at a three times greater risk of sustaining another TBI as compared with the general population.[72] As such, an important distal role of cognitive rehabilitation is to prevent substance abuse. This outcome has yet to be empirically demonstrated due to the need to follow individuals for many years following treatment termination.

Alarmingly high rates of TBI have been found among individuals who are homeless or incarcerated. One study conducted in homeless shelters and respite clinics found that 67% of homeless respondents reported a history of TBI, and of these, 71% reported having sustained more than one head injury.[74] Based on the age at injury (72% occurred before the age of 25), etiology of injuries (more than half were motor vehicle accidents, work-related injuries, or sports-related injuries), and recent timing of homelessness (72% had been homeless for <5 years), it appears that homelessness may more commonly be a consequence than a cause of TBI.[74] Similarly, several studies conducted involving individuals who are incarcerated have found that up to 87% of inmates report having experienced a TBI.[14,73] High rates of precrime TBI are also reported among juvenile offenders.[75,76]

To the extent that antisocial and self-injurious behaviors are consequences of untreated neurobehavioral symptoms, it may be true that cognitive rehabilitation can play an important role in their prevention. Indeed, the vast majority of homeless and incarcerated individuals with a history of TBI report not having received any kind of rehabilitation after their injuries.[74] When left untreated, over time, the multifaceted impairments that result from TBI contribute to reductions in psychosocial functioning and quality of life, and individuals with TBI are at elevated risk for experiencing myriad negative consequences.

SUMMARY

The literature provides a large body of evidence supporting the impact of cognitive rehabilitation on improving the cognitive, emotional, and behavioral functioning of individuals with TBI. Individuals may be referred to or seek cognitive rehabilitation for a variety of reasons. While measurement of rehabilitation outcomes is limited to those constructs for which psychometrically sound assessment instruments exist, clinicians commonly observe improvements in interpersonal relationships, increased confidence, and the capacity to create a meaningful and fulfilling life. Other potential roles of cognitive rehabilitation continue to be explored, such as the capacity to facilitate natural recovery with neuroplasticity-based cognitive interventions delivered during the acute phases of rehabilitation[77] or the use of Internet-based social networking tools to reduce social isolation and enhance vocational and personal networks.[78]

REFERENCES

1. Ashman TA, Gordon WA, Cantor JB, et al. Neurobehavioral consequences of traumatic brain injury. Mt Sinai J Med 2006;73(7):999–1005.
2. Dijkers MP. Quality of life after traumatic brain injury: a review of research approaches and findings. Arch Phys Med Rehabil 2004;85:S21–35.
3. Stratton MC, Gregory RJ. After traumatic brain injury: a discussion of consequences. Brain Inj 1995;8(7):631–45.
4. Brown M, Vandergoot D. Quality of life for individuals with traumatic brain injury: comparison with others living in the community. J Head Trauma Rehabil 1998; 13(4):1–23.
5. Ruff R. Two decades of advances in understanding of mild traumatic brain injury. J Head Trauma Rehabil 2005;20(1):5–18.
6. Gordon WA, Hibbard MR. Cognitive rehabilitation. In: Silver JM, Yudoffsky SC, McAllister TW, editors. Neuropsychiatry of traumatic brain injury. 2nd edition. Washington, DC: American Psychiatric Press; 2005. p. 655–60.
7. Lezak M, Howieson DB, Loring DW. Neuropsycological assessment. New York: Oxford University Press; 2004.
8. Silver JM, McAllister JW, Yudofsky SC. Textbook of traumatic brain injury. 1st edition. Washington, DC: American Psychiatric Publishing, Incorporated; 2005.
9. Consensus conference. Rehabilitation of persons with traumatic brain injury. NIH Consensus Development Panel on Rehabilitation of Persons with Traumatic Brain Injury. JAMA 1999;282:974–83.
10. Hibbard MR, Uysal S, Kepler K, et al. Axis I psychopathology in individuals with traumatic brain injury. J Head Trauma Rehabil 1998;13(4):24–39.

11. Hibbard MR, Rendon D, Charatz H, et al. CBT in individuals with traumatic brain injury. In: Freeman SM, Freeman A, editors. Cognitive behavior therapy in nursing practice. New York: Springer Publishing Co; 2005. p. 189–220.

12. Hibbard MR, Uysal S, Sliwinski M, et al. Undiagnosed health issues in individuals with traumatic brain injury living in the community. J Head Trauma Rehabil 1998; 13(4):47–57.

13. Sacks A, Fenske C, Gordon W, et al. Comorbidity of substance abuse and traumatic brain injury. J Dual Diagn 2009;5:404–17.

14. Slaughter B, Fann JR, Ehde D. Traumatic brain injury in a county jail population: prevalence, neuropsychological functioning and psychiatric disorders. Brain Inj 2003;17(9):731–41.

15. Ben-Yishay Y. DL. Cognitive remediation in traumatic brain injury: update and issues. Arch Phys Med Rehabil 1993;74(2):204–13.

16. Cicerone KD, Dahlberg C, Kalmar K, et al. Evidence-based cognitive rehabilitation: recommendations for clinical practice. Arch Phys Med Rehabil 2000;81(12): 1596–615.

17. Cicerone KD, Dahlberg C, Malec JF, et al. Evidence-based cognitive rehabilitation: updated review of the literature from 1998 through 2002. Arch Phys Med Rehabil 2005;86(8):1681–92.

18. Cicerone K, Levin H, Malec J, et al. Cognitive rehabilitation interventions for executive function: moving from bench to bedside in patients with traumatic brain injury. J Cogn Neurosci 2006;18(7):1212–22.

19. Cappa SF, Benke T, Clarke S, et al. EFNS guidelines on cognitive rehabilitation: report of an EFNS task force. Eur J Neurol 2003;10(1):11–23.

20. Kennedy MR, Coelho C, Turkstra L, et al. Intervention for executive functions after traumatic brain injury: a systematic review, meta-analysis and clinical recommendations. Neuropsychol Rehabil 2008;18(3):257–99.

21. Rohling ML, Faust ME, Beverly B, et al. Effectiveness of cognitive rehabilitation following acquired brain injury: a meta-analytic re-examination of Cicerone et al.'s (2000, 2005) systematic reviews. Neuropsychology 2009;23(1):20–39.

22. Sherer M, Roebuck-Spencer T, Davis LC. Outcome assessment in traumatic brain injury clinical trials and prognostic studies. J Head Trauma Rehabil 2010;25(2): 92–8.

23. Robertson IH, Murre JM. Rehabilitation of brain damage: brain plasticity and principles of guided recovery. Psychol Bull 1999;125(5):544–75.

24. Kasten E, Muller-Oehring E, Sabel BA. Stability of visual field enlargements following computer-based restitution training – results of a follow-up. J Clin Exp Neuropsychol 2001;23(3):297–305.

25. Serino A, Ciaramelli E, Santantonio AD, et al. A pilot study for rehabilitation of central executive deficits after traumatic brain injury. Brain Inj 2007;21(1):11–9.

26. Westerberg H, Jacobaeus H, Hirvikoski T, et al. Computerized working memory training after stroke—a pilot study. Brain Inj 2007;21(1):21–9.

27. Pulvermuller F, Neininger B, Elbert T, et al. Constraint-induced therapy of chronic aphasia after stroke. Stroke 2001;32(7):1621–6.

28. Meinzer M, Djundja D, Barthel G, et al. Long-term stability of improved language functions in chronic aphasia after constraint-induced aphasia therapy. Stroke 2005;36(7):1462–6.

29. Merzenich MM, Tallal P, Peterson B, et al. Some neurological principles relevant to the origins of—and the cortical plasticity-based remediation of—developmental language impairments. In: Grafman J, editor. Neuronal plasticity: building a bridge from the laboratory to the clinic. New York: Springer-Verlag; 1999. p. 169.

30. Mahncke HW, Bronstone A, Merzenich MM. Brain plasticity and functional losses in the aged: scientific bases for a novel intervention. Prog Brain Res 2006;157:81–109.

31. Lebowitz M, Dams-O'Connor K, Cantor J, et al. Examining the usability of a computerized cognitive training program in people with traumatic brain injury (TBI): a pilot study. Presented at the American Congress of Rehabilitation Medicine. Denver (CO), October 8, 2009.

32. Sohlberg MM, Avery J, Kennedy M, et al. Practice guidelines for direct attention training. J Med Speech Lang Pathol 2003;11(3):19–20, 29.

33. Tiersky LA, Anselmi V, Johnston MV, et al. A trial of neuropsychologic rehabilitation in mild-spectrum traumatic brain injury. Arch Phys Med Rehabil 2005;86(8):1565–74.

34. Poggel DA, Kasten E, Sabel BA. Attentional cueing improves vision restoration therapy in patients with visual field defects. Neurology 2004;63(11):2009–70.

35. Dams-O'Connor K. Strategy substitution. In: Kreutzer JS, DeLuca J, Caplan B, editors. Encyclopedia of clinical neurophyschology. Heidelberg (Germany): Springer; in press.

36. Fasotti L, Kovacs F, Eling PA, et al. Time pressure management as a compensatory strategy training after closed head injury. Neuropsychol Rehabil 2000;10(1):47–65.

37. Sohlberg MM, McLaughlin KA, Pavese A, et al. Evaluation of attention process training and brain injury education in persons with acquired brain injury. J Clin Exp Neuropsychol 2000;22(5):656–76.

38. Kaschel R, Della Sala S, Cantagallo A, et al. Imagery mnemonics for the rehabilitation of memory: a randomised group controlled trial. Neuropsychol Rehabil 2002;12(2):127–53.

39. Ownsworth TL, Mcfarland K. Memory remediation in long-term acquired brain injury: two approaches in diary training. Brain Inj 1999;13(8):605–26.

40. Wilson BA, Emslie H, Quirk K, et al. A randomized control trial to evaluate a paging system for people with traumatic brain injury. Brain Inj 2005;19(11):891–4.

41. Wilson BA, Emslie HC, Quirk K, et al. Reducing everyday memory and planning problems by means of a paging system: a randomised control crossover study. J Neurol Neurosurg Psychiatry 2001;70(4):477–82.

42. Ehlhardt LA, Sohlberg MM, Glang A, et al. A pilot study evaluating an instructional sequence for persons with impaired memory and executive functions. Brain Inj 2005;19(8):569–83.

43. Melton AK, Bourgeois MS. Training compensatory memory strategies via the telephone for persons with TBI. Aphasiology 2007;19:353–4.

44. Bourgeois MS, Lenius K, Turkstra L. The effects of cognitive teletherapy on reported everyday memory behaviours of persons with chronic traumatic brain injury. Brain Inj 2007;21(12):1245–57.

45. Rath JF, Simon D, Langenbahn DM, et al. Group treatment of problem-solving deficits in outpatients with traumatic brain injury: a randomized outcome study. Neuropsychol Rehabil 2003;13:341–88.

46. Hewitt J, Evans JJ, Dritschel B. Theory driven rehabilitation of executive functioning: improving planning skills in people with traumatic brain injury through the use of an autobiographical episodic memory cueing procedure. Neuropsychologia 2006;44(8):1468–74.

47. Levine B, Robertson IH, Clare L, et al. Rehabilitation of executive functioning: an experimental-clinical validation of goal management training. J Int Neuropsychol Soc 2000;6(3):299–312.

48. Ownsworth TL, McFarland K, Young RM. The investigation of factors underlying deficits in self-awareness and self-regulation. Brain Inj 2002;16(4):291–309.

49. Goverover Y, Johnston MV, Toglia J, et al. Treatment to improve self-awareness in persons with acquired brain injury. Brain Inj 2007;21(9):913–23.

50. Cheng SK, Man DW. Management of impaired self-awareness in persons with traumatic brain injury. Brain Inj 2006;20(6):621–8.

51. Ownsworth TL, McFarland KM, Young RM. Development and standardization of the self-regulation skills interview (SRSI): a new clinical assessment tool for acquired brain injury. Clin Neuropsychol 2000;14(1):76–92.

52. Fann JR, Bombardier CH, Temkin NR, et al. Incidence, severity, and phenomenology of depression and anxiety in patients with moderate to severe traumatic brain injury. Psychosomatics 2003;44:161.

53. Seel RT, Kreutzer JS, Rosenthal M, et al. Depression after traumatic brain injury: a national institute on disability and rehabilitation research model systems multicenter investigation. Arch Phys Med Rehabil 2003;84(2):177–84.

54. Fann JR, Hart T, Schomer KG. Treatment for depression after traumatic brain injury: a systematic review. J Neurotrauma 2009;26(12):2383–402.

55. Simpson G, Tate R. Suicidality in people surviving a traumatic brain injury: prevalence, risk factors and implications for clinical management. Brain Inj 2007;21:1335–51.

56. Silver JM, Kramer R, Greenwald S, et al. The association between head injuries and psychiatric disorders: findings from the new haven NIMH epidemiologic catchment area study. Brain Inj 2001;15:935–45.

57. Chen JK, Johnston KM, Petrides M, et al. Neural substrates of symptoms of depression following concussion in male athletes with persisting postconcussion symptoms. Arch Gen Psychiatry 2008;65(1):81–9.

58. Jorge RE, Robinson RG, Moser D, et al. Major depression following traumatic brain injury. Arch Gen Psychiatry 2004;61(1):42–50.

59. Beck AT, Rush AJ, Shaw BF, et al. Cognitive therapy of depression. New York: Guilford Press; 1979.

60. Hibbard MR, Bogdany J, Uysal S, et al. Axis II psychopathology in individuals with traumatic brain injury. Brain Inj 2000;14(1):45–61.

61. Medd J, Tate RL. Evaluation of an anger management therapy programme following ABI: a preliminary study. Neuropsychol Rehabil 2000;10:185.

62. Brooks N, McKinlay W, Symington C, et al. Return to work within the first seven years of severe head injury. Brain Inj 1987;1(1):5–19.

63. Temkin NR, Corrigan JD, Dikmen SS, et al. Social functioning after traumatic brain injury. J Head Trauma Rehabil 2009;24(6):460–7.

64. Yasuda S, Wehman P, Targett P, et al. Return to work for persons with traumatic brain injury. Am J Phys Med Rehabil 2001;80(11):852–64.

65. Kendall E, Muenchberger H, Gee T. Vocational rehabilitation following traumatic brain injury: a quantitative synthesis of outcome studies. J Vocat Rehabil 2006;25(3):149–60.

66. Wilson BA. Neuropsychological rehabilitation. Annu Rev Clin Psychol 2008;4:141–62.

67. Dahlberg CA, Cusick CP, Hawley LA, et al. Treatment efficacy of social communication skills training after traumatic brain injury: a randomized treatment and deferred treatment controlled trial. Arch Phys Med Rehabil 2007;88(12):1561–73.

68. McDonald S, Tate R, Togher L, et al. Social skills treatment for people with severe, chronic acquired brain injuries: a multicenter trial. Arch Phys Med Rehabil 2008;89(9):1648–59.

69. Ben-Yishay Y, Rattock J, Lakin P, et al. Silver sea. Neuropsychological rehabilitation: quest for a holistic approach. Semin Neurol 1985;5:252–8.
70. Cicerone KD, Mott T, Azulay J, et al. A randomized controlled trial of holistic neuropsychologic rehabilitation after traumatic brain injury. Arch Phys Med Rehabil 2008;89(12):2239–49.
71. Corrigan JD, Bogner JA. Neighborhood characteristics and outcomes after traumatic brain injury. Arch Phys Med Rehabil 2008;89(5):912–21.
72. Brain Injury Association of America. Substance abuse issues after traumatic brain injury. Available at: http://www.biausa.org/elements/BIAM/2004/substanceabuse.pdf2010. Accessed May 21, 2009.
73. Schofield PW, Butler TG, Hollis SJ, et al. Traumatic brain injury among Australian prisoners: rates, recurrence and sequelae. Brain Inj 2006;20(5):499–506.
74. Waldmann C, Roncaratl J, Swaln S, et al. Traumatic brain injury in the homeless population: incidence and impact. Presented at APHA 135th Annual Meeting and Expo: Politics, Policy, and Public Health. Washington, DC, November 3–7, 2007.
75. Leon-Carrion J, Ramos FJ. Blows to the head during development can predispose to violent criminal behaviour: rehabilitation of consequences of head injury is a measure for crime prevention. Brain Inj 2003;17(3):207–16.
76. Timonen M, Miettunen J, Hakko H, et al. The association of preceding traumatic brain injury with mental disorders, alcoholism and criminality: the northern Finland 1966 birth cohort study. Psychiatry Res 2002;113(3):217–26.
77. Dams-O'Connor K, Lebowitz M, Cantor JB, et al. Feasibility of a computerized cognitive skill-building program in an inpatient TBI rehabilitation setting. Presented at the American Congress of Rehabilitation Medicine. Denver (CO), October 8, 2009.
78. Tsaousides T, Lebowitz M, Matsuzawa Y, et al. Facebook use among individuals with brain injury: new opportunities for social integration. Presented at the 8th World Congress on Brain Injury. Washington, DC, March 10–14, 2010.

Personalized Medicine in Traumatic Brain Injury

Giulio Maria Pasinetti, MD, PhD[a,b,*], Hayley Fivecoat, BS[a],
Lap Ho, PhD[a]

KEYWORDS

- Postconcussive traumatic brain injury • MicroRNA • Biomarker
- Personalized medicine

A fine line exists between a trivial head blow and one that affects the brain to produce a mild traumatic brain injury (TBI). The widely varying clinical effects of mild brain injury provide grounds for substantial physical, cognitive, and psychosocial disability. To this end, an opinion may be requested of a rehabilitation specialist, neurologist, psychiatrist, or other physician seeing the patient for the first time months, or even years, after the traumatic event. Ideally, for an evidence-based diagnosis of a postconcussive disorder to be made, the following 4 factors are required: (1) a credible mechanistic force applied to the brain, sufficient to cause microstructural or at least molecular injury to the brain; (2) acute clinical effects that are both recognizable and verifiable; (3) partitioning of nonspecific or confounding symptoms and findings arising independently of the brain injury; and (4) a discernible end point of recovery or disability.[1] A strong need exists for the creation of minimum objective requirements and guidelines based on these precepts to determine whether a mild brain injury has occurred resulting in postconcussive symptoms. A second area in need of research is in establishing whether "persistent postconcussive syndrome" exists as a distinct biological entity. Yet a third area in need of research is in elucidating criteria that establish chronic traumatic encephalopathy as a unique cognitive disorder. As discussed in this article, these important questions may be addressed with the aid

This work was generously supported by the Department of Defense DM102029.

[a] Department of Neurology, Mount Sinai School of Medicine, One Gustave L. Levy Place, Box 1137, New York, NY 10029, USA

[b] Geriatric Research, Education and Clinical Center, James J. Peters Veteran Affairs Medical Center, 130 West Kingsbridge Road, Bronx, NY 10468, USA

* Corresponding author. Department of Neurology, Mount Sinai School of Medicine, One Gustave L. Levy Place, Box 1137, New York, NY 10029.
E-mail address: giulio.pasinetti@mssm.edu

of current genomic technologies providing selective molecular signatures of disease ahead of time before clinical symptoms become available.

TOWARD PERSONALIZED MEDICINE IN TBI

The identification and characterization of "molecular fingerprints" of postconcussive disorders is critical in establishing that symptoms are related to a mild TBI. Posttraumatic symptoms can develop in the hours and days after a mild TBI and may include insomnia, stress, headaches, pain, and mood disturbances.[1] The availability of mild TBI biomarkers offer a potential tool to ascertain that injury has occurred, and may provide a marker for prognosis and a guide for treatment response. Recent evidence identified microRNAs (miRNA) as important regulators of cellular function,[2,3] and that deregulation of select miRNA network in the brain has been associated with neurodegenerative disorders.[4-8] Moreover, there is accumulating evidence that supports the feasibility of using miRNA fingerprints from peripheral blood mononuclear cells (PBMC) to identify clinically accessible molecular indexes (biomarkers) of neurological disorders, with the potential for developing these biomarkers as practical diagnostic biological surrogates for the onset and clinical progression of a neurodegenerative disorder (see later discussion). Thus, it has been hypothesized that comparable strategies could be used to identify and characterize molecular indexes (biomarkers) capable of predicting the risk for the development of postconcussive symptoms or chronic traumatic encephalopathy (CTE). The development of specific biomarkers for mild TBI holds the potential to provide insights on novel strategies to prevent or minimize post-TBI sequelae.

An emerging health care challenge exists in the United States for how to best care for the increasingly large number of military veterans, particularly those involved in Operation Enduring Freedom and Operation Iraqi Freedom (OEF/OIF), who have been exposed to concussive injuries. The scientific development of molecular indexes that can signal complications of mild TBI, before the appearance of clinical signs and symptoms, is in line with the health care strategy of the United States Departments of Veteran Affairs and Defense, which focuses on prevention and early intervention rather than reactions to advanced stages of diseases.

LACK OF ESTABLISHED THERAPY FOR COMBAT-RELATED TBI

Based on the presumption that TBI induces structural brain damage and that recovery depends on adaptation, treatment of postconcussive symptoms to date has focused on pharmacotherapy to target individual symptoms, on cognitive rehabilitation mainly to help attention and memory, and on compensatory strategies through cognitive-behavioral therapies.[9] Although evidence supports the efficacy of cognitive-behavioral therapies for treating TBI in the civilian population,[10-13] many clinical trials have failed to reduce disability.[14,15] Moreover, no consensus exists on how to best treat combat-related TBI among OIF/OEF military personnel during and/or following their military deployment.

The mechanisms underlying mechanical and blast-related TBI may differ in some ways, but they share important pathophysiological features. Of note, a common feature of mechanical and blast injury is diffuse axonal injury caused by angular forces, which induce the shearing or stretching of axons.[9,16,17] This shearing results in impaired axonal transport and focal axonal swellings,[9] leading to impaired neurological functions. This and other similarities between the pathophysiologies of mechanical and blast-related TBI[9] suggest that information gathered from TBI in the civilian population may also be relevant to combat-related TBI.

VARIABLE SUSCEPTIBILITY OR RESILIENCY AMONG INDIVIDUALS EXPOSED TO MILD TBI

Mild TBI patients from both civilian and military populations exhibit varying clinical symptoms with minimal to profound impact on their daily functioning. This variation is reflected in a recently published mental health outcome survey of 105 OIF combatants diagnosed with mild TBI.[18] In this study, health status of eligible deployed military personnel was assessed by thorough review of their clinical records, and both diagnostic and injury severity scores were assigned.[19,20] Twenty-nine cases (27.6%) had presenting mental health problems (International Classification of Diseases [ICD-9] 290–319), with 17 out of the 29 cases presenting mood disorder (ICD-9 296, 300.4, 301.13, 311) and anxiety disorders (ICD-9 300–300.02, 300.21–300.29, 300.3, 308.3, 308.9, 309.81). Thus, clinical repercussions of mild TBI vary significantly among individuals.

The reason why mild TBI is associated with varying clinical symptoms among different individuals in response to mechanical or blast trauma among civilians or combat veterans is currently unknown. The possibility that miRNA from PBMC may reflect phenotypic changes in response to the mild TBI represents an unprecedented opportunity to explore the biomarker expressions that underlie the range of symptom expression observed after TBI.

POTENTIAL INTERRELATIONSHIPS BETWEEN TBI AND ALZHEIMER DISEASE–TYPE COGNITIVE DETERIORATION

Current literature suggests that TBI may be a risk factor for dementia and that they may be a cumulative risk from repeat events.[21] Although the early literature suggested that neuropathological mechanisms known to underlie Alzheimer disease (AD) dementia may have been similar to the one occurring in post-TBI patients, new evidence suggests that CTE is characterized by neuropathological findings that are distinct from the findings in AD.[22] The pathologic findings in these patients are believed to be responsible for cognitive decline seen in some patients with histories of TBI. The 2 characteristic neuropathologies of AD are the abnormal accumulation and deposition of beta-amyloid (Aβ) peptides and tau proteins in the brain. Evidence from humans[22–24] and experimental animal models[25] has also revealed abnormal accumulations of Aβ peptides and tau proteins in the brain and in cerebral spinal fluids following TBI; however, the location and the distribution of tau protein in TBI patients are different from the characteristic pattern seen in AD. Of note, there is some evidence suggesting that elevation of plasma tau levels has been associated with increasingly severe outcomes of TBI.[26] Thus, AD-related neuropathological mechanisms may contribute to cognitive dysfunction in TBI. Consistent with this, a recent study demonstrated that cognitive and motor deficits following TBI in experimental mouse models could be ameliorated by blocking either β- or γ-secretase, the 2 enzymes necessary for the generation of Aβ peptides from the amyloid precursor protein.[27] Molecular fingerprinting studies may lead to a better understanding of why certain individuals who have sustained a mild TBI may be susceptible to developing dementia.

FROM VISUAL PHENOTYPE TO HIDDEN MOLECULAR SIGNATURES: PERSONALIZED MEDICINE AND MILD TBI

In modern medicine, physicians and scientists alike have viewed and interpreted disease at the "visual" level, namely the level of the organism, the organ, and more recently, the tissue. With the advent of genomics and proteomics technologies, personalized medicine offers the promise and potential of uncovering the largely "unseen" details of disease causality, onset, and progression. A broad aim of personalized medicine is to use a molecular characterization approach to create a better system for disease classification. This work is anticipated to lead to earlier interventions and more specific treatments according to an individual's specific biochemical fingerprint; this is in stark contrast to current medical practice that is focused on the present state of health or disease. The differences between these 2 approaches may be best understood by likening them to one's view of an iceberg, which historically has been defined only by the very small part that is visible and almost inconsequential in relation to the predominant part that is below the surface yet defines the essence of the iceberg's existence (**Fig. 1**). Likewise, until now scientists and physicians have been limited to viewing and interpreting the most easily visible aspects of disease (at organism, organ, and tissue levels); by contrast, personalized medicine promises to reveal a far deeper and more comprehensive view of the largely unseen details of disease causality, onset, and progression by enabling them to view a disease from its onset and to monitor its progression at the molecular and cellular levels. Thus, the clinical presentations of patients who have sustained a mild TBI is conceptually comparable to the "tip of the iceberg" when the major impacts of the disease remain unseen. However, and most importantly, our understanding of disease is enhanced by the ability to view the "hidden, submerged unseen mass" of a given condition from its onset or, in other words, by the ability to monitor disease progression at the molecular level through the use of novel genomic technology (eg, miRNA at the cellular-molecular level, as depicted in **Fig. 1**). To date, some specific examples of personalized

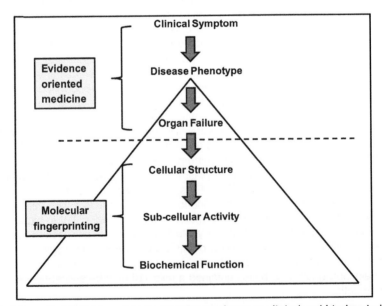

Fig. 1. Schematic subdivision of postconcussive syndrome as clinical and biochemical entity at various functional levels within an organism following mild TBI. The top bracket embraces those levels of disease for which traditional "evidence-oriented" medicine has been successful in the last 2 centuries (tip of the iceberg). The lower bracket embraces the extended region accessible by personalized medicine attempting to define the disease at cellular/biochemical levels.

medicine approaches, including the recent use of miRNA, have been utilized to benefit diagnosis and treatment of diseases in patients.

BIOLOGY OF miRNA AND THE SILENCING OF GENE EXPRESSION: IMPLICATIONS FOR UNDERSTANDING NEURODEGENERATIVE DISORDERS

The miRNA species are naturally present in 21- to 22-nucleotide base RNAs, functioning to silence their target genes' messenger RNAs either by binding to the coding region and promoting cleavage and degradation, or by inhibiting their translation by binding at the 3'-untranslated region (UTR).[28,29] New evidence points to miRNA as an important index of gene regulation.[2,3] An individual miRNA may target many gene transcripts that include specific target sequences; at the same time, a target gene's messenger RNA may possess multiple target sequences vulnerable to control by multiple miRNAs.[30] This versatility in miRNA silencing provides cells with an exquisite ability to programmatically shift rapidly among various signaling pathways. This exciting emerging discovery of the suppressing action of miRNAs does not negate the importance of other biological processes involved in controlling gene expression such as promoter-based transcriptional regulation, changes in DNA structure, or binding interaction to nuclear proteins. Most importantly, it serves as a complementary system to transcriptional control and modifying the intensity of individual gene expression in order to obtain a spectrum of its signal manifestation rather than an all-or-none outcome. miRNAs have recently emerged as key regulators of complex temporal and spatial patterns of gene/protein expression changes and, thereby, synaptic and neural plasticity.[28,31] Accumulating evidence suggests that selectively deregulated miRNA expression networks in the brain could mechanistically contribute to the onset and/or progression of neurodegenerative disorders, including AD,[4–6] Huntington disease,[7] and Parkinson disease.[8] These findings suggest that there are underlying genetic mechanisms that affect the brain's response to injury and, if true, would explain the individual variability in response to TBI.

EVIDENCE SUPPORTING THE FEASIBILITY OF USING CLINICALLY ACCESSIBLE MOLECULAR INDEXES FOR DEVELOPING PERSONALIZED MEDICINE APPROACHES IN MILD TBI PREVENTIVE STRATEGIES

There is increasing interest in exploring the prognostic values of plasma molecular signatures to predict clinical outcome following TBI. Indeed, high serum levels of S100B,[32] neuron-specific enolase,[32,33] glial fibrillary acidic protein,[32] and tau[26,34] following TBI have been linked to poor long-term outcome. Detecting abnormal levels of these markers may trigger interventions aimed at preventing future disease. Two genetic tests currently on the market can identify disease susceptibility and guide preventive care. First, a recent molecular predictive indicator of disease, which has received wide attention, is the test for BRCA1 and BRCA2, 2 genetic variants that indicate a hereditary propensity for breast and ovarian cancers.[35] Women with BRCA1 or BRCA2 genetic risk factors have a 36% to 85% lifetime chance of developing breast cancer, compared with a 13% chance among the general female population. The BRCA1 and BRCA2 genetic tests can be used to guide preventive measures, such as increased frequency of mammography, prophylactic surgery, and chemoprevention. Second, the treatment of early-stage breast cancer in women may be transformed, for example, by several assays in development that scan a panel of genes correlated with risk of disease recurrence and response to therapy.[36] One such assay now being used in clinical settings is Oncotype DX (Genomic Health, Redwood City, CA), which analyzes the expression of 21 genes.[37]

It can be hypothesized that similar approaches may soon be available for identifying patients at risk for developing postconcussive disorders including CTE. The information provided by such a test would be fundamental to supporting both disease treatment and monitoring decisions, based on the foreknowledge of disease progression, time to event, and likelihood of treatment benefit.[38] The degree of success in individualizing medicine in TBI and neuropsychological complications, however, will depend on the degree to which molecular aspects of the disease can be elucidated and measured. Feasibility studies of Parkinson disease suggest that miRNA technology holds the potential to provide a novel, clinically accessible tool for preventative medicine strategies in mild TBI (Pasinetti and Ho, personal Communication, 2008). The authors' laboratory has demonstrated for the first time that the regulation of specific peripheral molecular indices (eg, miRNA in PBMC) is associated with the onset and/ or progression of Parkinson disease. In recent ongoing studies, higher contents of 3 PBMC miRNA biomarkers have been found in the substantia nigra specimens of Parkinson patients than in normal cases. The authors' success in identifying peripheral biomarkers for Parkinson disease strongly supports the hypothesis that a comparable genomic technological approach could be used in the identification of biomarkers for the development of postconcussive disorders.

Thus, the use of high-throughput miRNA assays combined with reverse transcription–polymerase chain reaction validation studies might lead to the identification and characterization of molecular fingerprints (ie, biomarkers) associated with TBI phenotypic expression among individuals with mild TBI. These clinically accessible biomarkers provide the opportunity to test whether postconcussive symptoms of CTE could be predicted at molecular levels in patients with TBI prior to definitive clinical diagnosis.[1] Moreover, the availability of TBI biomarkers may provide a better understanding of the molecular mechanisms underlying resiliency to TBI clinical complications, and may provide predictive biomarkers of resiliency/susceptibility to TBI clinical complications. Ultimately, clinically accessible TBI biomarkers may provide the basis for developing a novel personalized medicine approach to the treatment of patients with mild TBI. Based on evidence from the authors' laboratory that miRNA species in PBMC may reflect neurodegenerative disorders (eg, Parkinson disease) at early, preclinical phases of the disease, it can be posited that PBMC may provide an ideal and clinically accessible "window" into the brain. Thus, it is possible that changes in the expression profile of clinically accessible biomarkers, such as miRNA in PBMC, may reflect molecular alterations following TBI that contribute to the onset and progression of TBI phenotypes.

SUMMARY: IMPACT OF THE CLINICALLY ACCESSIBLE BIOMARKERS IN MILD TBI

According to existing data, more than 1.5 million people are treated in hospitals for TBI each year in the United States, 75% of whom for mild TBI.[38] These injuries may cause long-term or permanent impairments and disabilities. Many people with mild TBI have difficulty returning to routine, daily activities and may be unable to return to work for many weeks or months. In addition to the human toll of these injuries, mild TBI costs the nation nearly $17 billion each year.[38] These data, however, likely underestimate the problem of mild TBI for several reasons: first, no standard definitions exist for mild TBI and mild TBI-related impairments and disabilities. The existing Centers for Disease Control and Prevention (CDC) definition for TBI surveillance is designed to identify cases of TBI that result in hospitalization, which tend to be more severe. Mild TBI is often treated in nonhospital settings, or is not treated at all. Few states conduct emergency department–based surveillance, and current efforts do not capture data about persons with mild TBI who receive no medical treatment. In addition, neither hospital-based nor emergency department–based data can provide estimates of the long-term consequences of mild TBI. In response to concerns about this public health problem, Congress passed the Children's Health Act of 2000, which required the CDC to determine how best to measure the incidence (ie, rate at which new cases of mild TBI occur) and the prevalence (ie, proportion of the United States population at any given time that is experiencing the effects) of mild TBI, and to report the findings to Congress.[39,40] To that end, the CDC formed the Mild Traumatic Brain Injury Work Group to determine appropriate and feasible methods for assessing the incidence and prevalence of mild TBI in the United States.

The development of clinically accessible biomarkers, such as specific miRNA biomarker species in PBMC, will serve as independent, objective biological surrogates to help predict complications of TBI in a population (such as veterans who sustained a concussive injury) at high risk for developing postconcussive disorders. This particular aim is in line with the Children's Health Act of 2000 and CDC mission. This new approach will make it possible to use molecular indexes that signal the risk of developing postconcussive sequelae or its presence before clinical signs and symptoms appear, and has the potential to have a major impact in preventative measures among combat veterans and in the American civilian public sector.

REFERENCES

1. Rees PM. Contemporary issues in mild traumatic brain injury. Arch Phys Med Rehabil 2003;84:1885–94.
2. Cai Y, Yu X, Hu S, et al. A brief review on the mechanisms of miRNA regulation. Genomics Proteomics Bioinformatics 2009;7:147–54.
3. Takacs CM, Firaldez AJ. MicroRNAs as genetic sculptors: fishing for clues. Semin Cell Dev Biol 2010;21(7):760–7.
4. Wang WX, Rajeev BW, Stromberg AJ, et al. The expression of microRNA miR-107 decreases early in Alzheimer's disease and may accelerate disease progression through regulation of beta-site amyloid precursor protein-cleaving enzyme 1. J Neurosci 2008;28:1213–23.
5. Hebert SS, Horre K, Nicolai L, et al. Loss of microRNA cluster miR-29a/b-1 in sporadic Alzheimer's disease correlates with increased BACE1/beta-secretase expression. Proc Natl Acad Sci U S A 2008;105:6415–20.
6. Shioya M, Obayashi S, Tabunoki H, et al. Aberrant microRNA expression in the brains of neurodegenerative diseases: miR-29a decreased in Alzheimer disease brains targets neuron navigator-3. Neuropathol Appl Neurobiol 2010;36:320–30.
7. Packer AN, Xing Y, Harper SQ, et al. The bifunctional microRNA miR-9/miR-9* regulates REST and CoREST and is down-regulated in Huntington's disease. J Neurosci 2008;28:14341–6.
8. Kim J, Inoue K, Ishii J, et al. A MicroRNA feedback circuit in midbrain dopamine neurons. Science 2007;317:1220–4.
9. Elder GA, Cristian A. Blast-related mild traumatic brain injury: mechanisms of injury and impact on clinical care. Mt Sinai J Med 2009;76:111–8.
10. Cappa SF, Benke T, Clarke S, et al. EFNS guidelines on cognitive rehabilitation: report of an EFNS task force. Eur J Neurol 2005;12:665–80.
11. Chua KS, Ng YS, Yap SG, et al. A brief review of traumatic brain injury rehabilitation. Ann Acad Med Singap 2007;36:31–42.
12. Cicerone KD. Evidence-based cognitive rehabilitation: updated review of the literature from 1998 through 2002. Arch Phys Med Rehabil 2005;86:1681–92.

13. Geusgens CA, Winkens I, van Heugten CM, et al. Occurrence and measurement of transfer in cognitive rehabilitation: a critical review. J Rehabil Med 2007;39: 425–39.
14. Gordon WA, Zafonte R, Cicerone K, et al. Traumatic brain injury rehabilitation: state of the science. Am J Phys Med Rehabil 2006;85:343–82.
15. Saatman KE, Duhaime AC, Bullock R, et al. Classification of traumatic brain injury for targeted therapies. J Neurotrauma 2008;25:719–38.
16. Lux WE. A neuropsychiatric perspective on traumatic brain injury. J Rehabil Res Dev 2007;44:951–62.
17. Orrison WW, Hanson EH, Alamo T, et al. Traumatic brain injury: a review and high-field MRI findings in 100 unarmed combatants using a literature-based checklist approach. J Neurotrauma 2009;26:689–701.
18. MacGregor AJ, Shaffer RA, Dougherty AL, et al. Prevalence and psychological correlates of traumatic brain injury in Operation Iraqi Freedom. J Head Trauma Rehabil 2010;25:1–8.
19. Ommaya AK, Ommaya AK, Dannenberg AL, et al. Causation, incidence, and costs of traumatic brain injury in the U.S. Military medical system. J Trauma 1996;40:211–7.
20. Gennarelli T, Wodzon E. The abbreviated injury scale—2005. Des Plaines (IL): Association for the Advancement of Automotive Medicine; 2005.
21. Van Duijn C, Tanja TA, Haaxma R, et al. Head trauma and the risk of Alzheimer's disease. Am J Epidemiol 1992;135:775–82.
22. McKee A, Cantu R, Nowinski C, et al. Chronic traumatic encephalopathy: progressive tauopathy after repetitive head injury. J Neuropathol Exp Neurol 2009;68:709–35.
23. Marklund N, Blennow K, Zetterberg H, et al. Monitoring of brain interstitial total tau and beta amyloid proteins by microdialysis in patients with traumatic brain injury. J Neurosurg 2009;110:1227–37.
24. Olsson A, Csajbok L, Ost M, et al. Marked increase of beta-amyloid(1-42) and amyloid precursor protein in ventricular cerebrospinal fluid after severe traumatic brain injury. J Neurol 2004;251:870–6.
25. Szczygielski J, Mautes A, Steudel WI, et al. Traumatic brain injury: cause or risk of Alzheimer's disease? A review of experimental studies. J Neural Transm 2005; 112:1547–64.
26. Liliang PC, Liang CL, Weng HC, et al. Tau proteins in serum predict outcome after severe traumatic brain injury. J Surg Res 2010;160:302–7.
27. Loane DJ, Pocivavsek A, Moussa CE, et al. Amyloid precursor protein secretases as therapeutic targets for traumatic brain injury. Nat Med 2009;15:377–9.
28. Gao FB. Posttranscriptional control of neuronal development by microRNA networks. Trends Neurosci 2008;31:20–6.
29. Griffiths-Jones S, Saini HK, van Dongen S, et al. miRBase: tools for microRNA genomics. Nucleic Acids Res 2008;36(Database issue):D154–8.
30. Breving K, Esquela-Kerscher A. The complexities of microRNA regulation: mirandering around the rules. Int J Biochem Cell Biol 2010;42(8):1316–29.
31. Schratt G. MicroRNAs at the synapse. Nat Rev Neurosci 2009;10:842–9.
32. Vos PE, Lamers KJ, Hendriks JC, et al. Glial and neuronal proteins in serum predict outcome after severe traumatic brain injury. Neurology 2004;62: 1303–10.
33. Bandyopadhyay S, Hennes H, Gorelick MH, et al. Serum neuron-specific enolase as a predictor of short-term outcome in children with closed traumatic brain injury. Acad Emerg Med 2005;12:732–8.

34. Zemlan FP, Jauch EC, Mulchahey JJ, et al. C-tau biomarker of neuronal damage in severe brain injured patients: association with elevated intracranial pressure and clinical outcome. Brain Res 2002;947:131–9.

35. Nelson HD, Huffman LH, Fu R, et al. Genetic risk assessment and BRCA mutation testing for breast and ovarian cancer susceptibility: systematic evidence review for the U.S. Preventive Services Task Force. Ann Intern Med 2005;143:362–79.

36. Paik S, Shak S, Tang G, et al. A multigene assay to predict recurrence of tamoxifen-treated, node-negative breast cancer. N Engl J Med 2004;351:2817–26.

37. Hornberger J, Cosler LE, Lyman GH. Economic analysis of targeting chemotherapy using a 21-gene RT-PCR assay in lymph-node-negative, estrogen-receptor-positive, early-stage breast cancer. Am J Manag Care 2005;11:313–22.

38. Paik S, Shak S, Tang G, et al. Gene expression and benefit of chemotherapy in women with node-negative, estrogen receptor-positive breast cancer. J Clin Oncol 2006;24:3726–34.

39. Greberding JL. Report to congress on mild traumatic brain injury in the United States: steps to prevent a serious public health problem. Centers for Disease Control and Prevention; 2003. Available at: http://www.cdc.gov/ncipc/pub-res/mtbi/mtbireport.pdf.

40. Berube JE. The Traumatic Brain Injury Act Amendments of 2000. J Head Trauma Rehabil 2001;16:210–3.

Current Issues in Neurolaw

Shana De Caro, Esq*, Michael V. Kaplen, Esq

KEYWORDS

- Traumatic brain injury • Neurologic rehabilitation
- Cognitive assessment

With the dramatic increase in attention on traumatic brain injury (TBI) by science, government, and the popular media, a subspecialty of the legal community focusing on issues related to neurologic care and outcomes, "neurolaw," has taken on correspondingly enhanced importance in the legal system. The brain is being placed on trial with increasing frequency in courtrooms throughout the nation encompassing a multitude of issues including:

- Injury reduction and prevention
- Evidentiary standards for the admissibility of expert testimony
- Competing definitions of mild traumatic brain injury and concussion
- Differentiating the persistent vegetative state from the minimally conscious state
- Emergency department assessments
- Forensic evaluations
- Cognitive evaluations and rehabilitation
- Disability and reimbursement controversies.

Addressing these issues within the context of the adversarial system, the legal profession must seek substantiation from medical science to corroborate a particular position or outcome. By necessity, attorneys must authenticate their arguments by reliance on scientific opinion on which there is often a lack of unanimity, within the (scientific) medical community. Even basic principles are awash in a contradictory body of literature, and in many cases are not borne out by evidence-based studies.

As a result of the increases in the number of individuals diagnosed with brain injury and the long-term survivability of individuals following brain trauma, the forensic aspects of TBI has taken on greater importance for both providers and patients. Increasingly successful medical interventions have led to greater attention on long-term outcome. The goal of this article is to highlight the major areas of controversy in TBI litigation that require synchronous resolution of both legal and medical issues.

De Caro & Kaplen LLP, 427 Bedford Road, Pleasantville, NY 10570, USA
* Corresponding author.
E-mail address: shana@brainlaw.com

Psychiatr Clin N Am 33 (2010) 915–930
doi:10.1016/j.psc.2010.09.002

It is imperative that neuroscience practitioners are conversant in these subjects and their ramifications from both perspectives, and are prepared to clarify them.

PREVALENCE

Trauma is the leading cause of brain injury in the United States, and leads to the inevitable involvement of the legal profession to mediate some of its consequences. According to the Centers for Disease Control and Prevention (CDC), TBI has become a national health epidemic[1]: the CDC reports that at least 1.7 million Americans seek hospital-based care for a TBI each year. Of those individuals about 52,000 die, 275,000 are hospitalized, and 1.365 million are treated and released from an emergency department (ED). The number of individuals who are not seen in a hospital and receive no care after sustaining a TBI is not currently known.

The major risk factors affecting TBI are age, gender, and low socioeconomic status. There is a higher rate of brain trauma in males (twice as high as females), which has been attributed to males' propensity for higher risk-taking behavior.[2] By event, falls are the leading cause of TBI (35.2%). Rates for falls are highest in children aged 0 to 4 years and for adults aged 75 years and older. Falls result in the greatest number of TBI-related ED visits (523,043) and hospitalizations (62,334). Motor vehicle accidents are the second leading cause of TBI (17.3%). Motor vehicle traffic injury is the leading cause of TBI-related death. Rates are highest in adults aged 20 to 24 years. Assaults account for 10%, which includes domestic violence, and is the third leading cause of all TBIs.

Epidemiologic analyses fail to capture the full extent of the burgeoning public health crisis from TBI, as many cases of brain trauma are unreported and therefore uncounted, especially in cases of domestic violence and sports concussions. Many of these individuals are never seen in EDs, and when treated, current criteria for brain assessment fail to include these patients. This systemic breakdown has far-reaching implications as it relates to health care planning and determining societal needs for prevention initiatives, acute assessment resources, and long-term rehabilitative services.

TRAUMATIC BRAIN INJURY IN THE COURTROOM

The contested issues of brain injury are seen through the prism of legal rules that govern the admissibility of evidence in the courtroom. The rules of evidence provide the guidelines for the introduction of both fact and opinion testimony during the course of a trial. The ultimate decision, usually by a jury, must be based on what has actually been introduced as evidence in the trial. In federal courts throughout the nation there is uniformity in the standards of evidence, in both civil and criminal proceedings, which are memorialized in the Federal Rules of Evidence. Although the Federal Rules do not apply to legal proceedings in state courts, the rules of most states are closely modeled after these provisions.

Federal Rule of Evidence (FRE) #104 states that the initial judicial inquiry as to the admissibility of any opinion evidence requires an examination of the qualifications of the person whose testimony is sought.[3] In the case of an expert witness, the threshold question is whether the expert has sufficient qualifications, by virtue of his or her knowledge, skill, experience, training, or education, to render an opinion. Thereafter, the inquiry proceeds to whether (1) the opinion is based on sufficient facts or data, (2) the testimony is the product of reliable principles and methods, and (3) the witness has applied scientific principles and methods reliably to the facts of the case. According to FRE #402, the evidence itself must be "relevant" to the issue ultimately to be decided. "Relevant evidence" means evidence having a tendency to make the existence of any fact that is of consequence to the determination of the action more or less probable than it would be without the evidence.

PRELIMINARY LEGAL CONSIDERATIONS FOR ADMISSIBILITY OF EXPERT TESTIMONY

There are a multitude of medical professionals whose opinions are typically used by attorneys litigating TBI cases, including neurologists, psychiatrists, rehabilitation medicine specialists, and radiologists. The opinions of professionals without a medical degree, such as neuropsychologists, are also frequently relied upon. Experts possessing medical degrees have traditionally been given wide latitude to render opinions, by virtue of their training and experience, concerning both the existence and cause of an injury, often referred to in legal parlance as the proximate or competent producing cause. Neurologists, psychiatrists, and rehabilitation specialists are often called on to render expert opinions based on their examination and treatment of injured claimants. Because of the interest of the legal profession in establishing "objective" evidence of brain damage, the assistance of neuroradiologists will become more prevalent and necessary as more objective tests of brain function are improved and developed.

Medical professionals operate as teachers in the courtroom, explaining to the finder of fact (usually a jury composed of 6 to 12 lay individuals) the structure and functioning of the brain, the manner in which brain damage takes place, and the physical, cognitive, behavioral, and social consequences of TBI. If they have also rendered professional care and treatment, they will explain the nature and extent of that treatment, as well as their diagnosis and prognosis for the patient. Frequently insurance carriers retain experts as well. These experts may comment on their examination of the claimant, their review of the plaintiff's medical records, the necessity of the treatment rendered, the accuracy of diagnosis, and the extent and permanency of injury and impairment; they may further proffer opinions as to alternative causes of the plaintiff's complaints. Forensic neuropsychiatrists will increasingly be called on to perform forensic assessments and answer specific psychiatric/legal questions using their unique training, experience, and methodology.

There are no specific legal qualifications for medical professionals in general, although various specialty societies have established their own guidelines for forensic evaluations and testimony. In the practice of neurology, forensic guidelines have been established by the American Academy of Neurology (AAN).[4] These guidelines provide, in part, that the expert neurologist should carefully and thoroughly review relevant medical and scientific data before offering an opinion. If the expert believes that the information provided is inaccurate or incomplete, he or she should refrain from rendering an opinion until the request for relevant data has met with compliance. The expert should be an active clinician if offering an expert opinion, and if not, should be prepared to demonstrate competence to provide the requested opinion. Competency to testify in this regard may be established by publication of relevant medical literature or active teaching in 3 of the previous past 5 years. Moreover, medical-legal activities, in general, should be limited to a maximum of 20% of the expert's professional time; if greater, the professional must be prepared to demonstrate that his or her testimony is not biased by financial considerations.

THE ROLE OF NEUROPSYCHOLOGISTS

Clinical neuropsychology has been defined as "an applied science concerned with the behavioral expression of brain dysfunction."[5] Neuropsychologists are often called on to provide neuropsychological evaluations in legal proceedings based on their interpretation of neuropsychological test results. The role of the neuropsychologist and use of neuropsychological testing has been endorsed by the AAN.[6] These test results are indispensable in establishing the existence and extent of TBI in the courtroom. General guidelines for the conduct of neuropsychological assessments can be found in the Practice Guidelines for the American Academy of Clinical Neuropsychology (AACN).[7] The extent to which these general guidelines can be applied, in the context of a forensic evaluation, and the need for the establishment of specific standards for forensic evaluations has been the subject of considerable debate.[8] While the test results themselves play a critical role in "neurolaw," there are no agreed-upon benchmarks for the conduct of a forensic neuropsychological assessment. The ethical principles established by the American Psychological Association (APA) specify that before a forensic psychological opinion is proffered, the psychologist should conduct a face-to-face examination of the individual involved.[9] If such an examination is not performed, the psychologist must document his or her efforts to conduct such an examination, and the limits and validity of his or her opinion, based on the failure to have performed this crucial evaluation.

The trial of a TBI case requires proof not only of an injury but also proof, through the opinion of a competent expert, that a specific event was the cause of the injury. The medical profession endorses the role and function of neuropsychologists and neuropsychological testing to establish the injury.[10] Most state courts allow causation testimony by neuropsychologists.[11] However, a minority of state courts reject the neuropsychologists' competence as to issues of causation; their lack of medical degrees is the basis for this testimonial limitation.[12] The courts in several states have ruled that the subject of causation and prognosis are peculiarly medical in nature, and require the testimony of a licensed physician.[13] Other states have ruled that the lack of a medical license does not, in and of itself, disqualify a witness from testifying as an expert on a medical question so long as the witness establishes that he or she is qualified by observation, experience, and/or academic study.[14]

SCIENTIFIC RELIABILITY

After the resolution of expert qualifications, the Court must act as a gatekeeper to determine whether the proposed testimony is scientifically reliable and therefore admissible. There are 2 alternative standards, depending on the jurisdiction, used to assess the reliability of scientific testimony. The traditional standard, known as the Frye standard, requires the Court to determine whether the testimony is based on an established scientific theory, and whether the techniques and decision-making processes are generally accepted within the scientific community.[15] Under a more modern standard, the Daubert standard (used in all Federal courts and increasingly in State Courts), judges must assess whether the expert's theory or technique has been tested, has been subjected to peer review, the known or potential rate of error, and whether the methodology is generally accepted in the field of inquiry.[16] The 3 primary sources of information that are most often used to formulate opinions as to brain injury are neuropsychological evidence, neuroradiological findings, and observations from friends, family, and coworkers: These 3 sources do not always support the same conclusion.[17]

Experts often encounter challenges to their opinions on the very existence of brain injury, based on questions concerning the reliability of neuropsychological testing and functional neuroimaging studies on which they rely. These objections often result in protracted court hearings with expert testimony elicited by both sides, and the introduction into evidence of conflicting scientific literature. Flexible neuropsychological test batteries have achieved general scientific acceptance and are most commonly used in forensic assessments. Only 15% of neuropsychologists reportedly use a fixed battery in forensic examinations.[18] The individual tests that compromise the test battery must each qualify as admissible, and the neuropsychologist must be prepared, if necessary, to establish that the individual tests meet the aforesaid standards of scientific reliability and acceptance, and that opinions derived therefrom are scientifically validated.[19]

Reliance on neuropsychological testing alone is insufficient to completely resolve the questions of whether an individual has sustained a TBI and the extent of that injury. Research supports the proposition that many individuals may perform satisfactorily on traditional neuropsychological testing and yet have difficulty with everyday decision making, and fail to do well in an unstructured environment or situation.[17] Moreover, this testing fails to address the important day-to-day dilemmas facing victims of brain injury. It is imperative that the testimony of the individual, friends, workers, and often disinterested coworkers be elicited to establish the day-to-day struggles and predicaments with which these individuals are confronted.

Imaging studies, such as positron emission tomography (PET) scans, diffusion tensor magnetic resonance imaging (DTI) studies, and functional MRI studies, have been subject to judicial scrutiny, with inconsistent rulings on their admissibility. The judicial hearings held to determine the admissibility of these studies typically focus on: (1) the presence or absence of acceptable norms or control groups, (2) evidence tending to establish whether the particular study has achieved general scientific acceptance in the field of TBI, (3) whether the test can validly detect brain damage in an individual, and (4) whether an expert can opine that an impairment can be linked to a specific outside event. As these imaging studies continue to gain acceptance in the scientific community, it can be anticipated that favorable court rulings will continue to proliferate.

WHAT IS MILD TRAUMATIC BRAIN INJURY?

Questions surrounding mild TBI generate the most attention and controversy in the legal realm. The debate concerning this condition finds origin in the dissonance in the medical profession concerning both the definition and diagnosis. There is friction regarding the assessment of behavioral and psychiatric issues, and disputes as to the long-term consequences. A jury's acceptance of mild TBI in a contested legal proceeding has the potential to result in substantial compensation of the victim, and therefore has particular significance to the legal profession.

The evidentiary issues facing victim and counsel in a mild TBI case are magnified, due to the "invisible" aspects of this injury to the unenlightened observer. The defense in many of these cases seems plausible because the individual appears normal, was not rendered unconscious, did not sustain any physical injuries, had a normal ED examination including a gross neurological evaluation, and had normal standard imaging studies.

Although many professional organizations have attempted to construct a working definition of mild TBI, these endeavors have been thwarted by the ongoing controversy concerning the relative importance of loss of consciousness and amnesia. Most current definitions of mild TBI include periods of observed or self-reported confusion or disorientation; however, the precise definition of these components is also subject to much conflict.[20] The event that gives rise to the injury is often unwitnessed, resulting in the absence of credible, immediate, on the scene observations regarding transient loss of consciousness, disorientation, and confusion. When emergency personnel arrive, the victim is often found walking and talking, and therefore the emergency responder may erroneously mistake such conduct for the absence of confusion, disorientation, or loss of consciousness. Because the victim is often asked questions he or she is incapable of answering accurately, issues of unconsciousness and posttraumatic amnesia are misunderstood. Asking the victim, "did you lose consciousness?" will not elicit a meaningful response.

Inherent in any definition of mild TBI is trauma of some sort. However, the amount, direction, or type of force required to produce this injury has not been settled. Both direct and indirect forces have been implicated in precipitating mild TBI and moreover, the consequences of rotational forces have recently received increased attention. On the battlefield, the Defense and Veterans Brain Injury Center (DVBIC) has acknowledged the limitations of current definitions in attempting to understand the physiological changes that take place following a blast injury, and have concluded that it is impossible to establish an absolute threshold for the establishment of a brain injury.[21]

If the information necessary to establish a diagnosis of mild TBI is missed at the scene of an accident, the next opportunity for the correct diagnosis to be made is typically in an ED. Unfortunately, even when a patient reports symptoms that indicate mild TBI the appropriate diagnosis may still not be made, as emergency physicians are focused on confirming brain pathology by computed tomography (CT) studies and questions of loss of consciousness. In one study, 56% of patients identified by a detailed examination of medical records as having the symptoms of mild TBI failed to receive that diagnosis on discharge.[22] Positive evidence of loss of consciousness produced greatest concurrence of opinion between researchers and emergency physicians, whereas a patient's reported confusion produced the greatest disagreement between researchers and emergency physicians as to the diagnosis of mild TBI.[23]

The search for objective evidence to substantiate the mild TBI often turns into a courtroom battle over the presence or absence of positive imaging studies. There is almost complete unanimity of medical opinion that the absence of positive imaging findings in CT studies and MRI studies is inconclusive as to the existence of brain injury. However, this offers little assistance to jurors who are searching for positive proof of injury, or to attorneys seeking positive confirmation of their client's symptoms and complaints. Newer imaging modalities such as PET scans, diffusion tensor imaging studies, and functional MRI studies have intensified attention on neuroradiological detection and objective confirmation of mild TBI, and may offer further guidance to both the court and jurors.

THE PERSISTENT VEGETATIVE STATE VERSUS THE MINIMALLY CONSCIOUS STATE

New research reexamining the accuracy of the diagnosis of persistent vegetative state has profound implications for attorneys seeking compensation for victims of severe TBI. Often patients are misdiagnosed as being in a persistent vegetative state, when in reality they are in a minimally conscious state. The minimally conscious state, distinguished from the vegetative state, is one in which the individual has severe alterations in consciousness, with minimal but definite behavioral evidence of self or environmental awareness.[24] Among the category of legal damage to which those in an impaired state of consciousness may be entitled are compensation for pain and suffering, and compensation for the loss of enjoyment of the pleasures and pursuits of life. The former is intended to compensate for what the injured individual must now endure, whereas the latter is intended to compensate for what was taken away or lost as a result of an injury. Many states, including New York, require proof of some type of conscious awareness before damages can be awarded for pain and suffering, or for the loss of the pleasures and pursuits of life.[25]

The diagnosis of persistent vegetative state will deprive the injured individual of the ability to obtain compensation for losses in jurisdictions that require some degree of conscious awareness. Estimates of misdiagnosis range from 15% to 43%.[26] Attempts to infer thought from observable behavior often proves unreliable. Misdiagnosis occurs as a result of the absence of absolute criteria to measure consciousness, and must depend solely on subjective determinations by observers as well as ambiguous and inconsistent responses made by the patient.[27] In patients with severe brain injury, the attempt to discern meaningful behavior is extremely difficult and prone to error.[28]

The challenge for clinicians and attorneys alike is to find some way of objectively determining whether an individual suffering from an impairment of consciousness has some degree of awareness. New medical research using functional MRI studies kindles the hope that this issue can now be addressed with a greater degree of accuracy. These studies have demonstrated, contrary to the impressions and evaluations of clinicians, that when those who had previously been diagnosed as in a persistent vegetative state were reassessed using functional MRI technology, some awareness and cognition was found to exist.[23]

EMERGENCY DEPARTMENT IMAGING IN MILD TRAUMATIC BRAIN INJURY

The tragic circumstances surrounding recently reported deaths of notable individuals raises important questions concerning medical assessment of what initially might not appear to be a TBI. Of course, before there can be an ED evaluation, someone must recognize the potential for significant brain trauma and make arrangements for the transport of the injured individual with potential brain damage to an ED capable of performing such an evaluation. This recognition requires the education of potential observers, especially in the sports arena, to recognize the signs and symptoms of brain trauma, to ask the appropriate questions, and to take appropriate and immediate steps to ensure proper evaluation.

Often unanswered questions linger concerning (1) the evaluation of the significance of a fall; (2) whether the individual struck his or her head; (3) if there was any period of unconsciousness or disorientation; (4) complaints the patient may have made at the scene including headaches, dizziness, nausea, and sensitivity to light or sound; and (5) any period of amnesia. Once in the hands of medical personnel, the law recognizes a cause of action in malpractice for the failure to diagnose a condition capable of diagnosis, if care was not rendered in accordance with good and proper medical protocol.[1] Liability can be imposed if the finder of fact determines that omissions and failure of care deprived the victim of a substantial possibility for a better outcome.[29]

In cases of mild TBI, decisions must be made in the ED to identify individuals who have sustained potentially significant intracranial injury, which may require neurosurgical intervention. To aid in this endeavor, the American College of Emergency Physicians has created practice guidelines for the use of noncontrast head CT scan in the management of adult mild TBI patients in the ED.[30] Attorneys seek to use clinical guidelines and standards to either establish conformity with or departure from the relevant standard of care. The admission into evidence of these guidelines and standards has significant implications for plaintiffs and defendants in medical malpractice cases; however, the rules concerning admissibility vary from jurisdiction to jurisdiction.[31,32] If admitted, these guidelines have the potential of becoming the focal point for the determination of whether there was a departure from good and accepted medical conduct.

PRESENCE OF THIRD-PARTY OBSERVERS DURING FORENSIC EVALUATIONS

A standard part of civil litigation is the compulsory examinations of claimants by medical personnel selected by defendants and used in actions for personal injury, workers' compensation evaluations, short- or long-term disability determinations, and automobile no-fault claims. These examinations, referred to as "Independent

Medical Examinations" by defense attorneys or "Insurance Medical Examinations" by plaintiff attorneys, are frequently conducted by neurologists, psychiatrists, neuropsychiatrists, psychologists, and neuropsychologists. Each side ascribes different motives and connotations to the examiners and their findings. The nomenclature reflects both the great reliance placed on them by defense attorneys and the great distrust that these examinations generate in plaintiffs' attorneys. Therefore, the integrity of the examination and their conclusions take on added significance in the courtroom, when the examiner must present his or her findings and conclusions.

In civil jurisprudence, there has been almost universal acceptance of the right of the claimant's attorney to be present and observe third-party mental and physical examinations. The right of attendance is premised on the presumption that these examinations are inherently adversarial in nature, and that an attorney has the right to be present to protect the interests of his or her client, to ensure the integrity of the examination, and to properly prepare for cross-examination. This right of observation has been codified in the Code of Civil Procedure in many states.[33] In some jurisdictions the right to transcribe or record the examination has also been permitted, whereas in others, videotaping of psychiatric examinations has been disallowed by the Court, although the presence of a stenographer outside of the room has been permitted.[34] Court decisions in New York State preclude the videotaping of a psychiatric examination based on the proposition that counsel for the plaintiff may be present to protect the plaintiff's rights,[35] but have allowed a stenographer to be outside of the room.[36]

In most TBI cases, the defense will retain the services of a neuropsychologist to conduct his or her own neuropsychological evaluation, as well as a psychiatrist or neuropsychiatrist to perform psychiatric evaluations. Issues concerning the manner in which the evaluation and testing was conducted, the way in which questions were presented, and the manner and accuracy of the recorded answers frequently arise. Attorneys handling these types of cases increasingly seek the right to retain an expert with the requisite training to observe and monitor the testing and examination, recognizing the need to verify their legitimacy and accuracy.

The demand to have a knowledgable third party present during these examinations has been subject to numerous and contradictory court decisions, determined on a state-by-state basis. The ruling hinges on the ability or inability to demonstrate that the third-party observer will, or potentially could, influence the outcome of the examination. For example, 2 recent New York State appellate decisions have held that in the case of neuropsychological examinations, plaintiffs had the right to be examined in the presence of their attorney or an observer chosen by their attorney, so long as that party did not interfere with the conduct of the examination, absent a showing by defense counsel that the presence of the third-party observer would "impair the validity and effectiveness" of the examination.[37]

The National Academy of Neuropsychology (NAN) has stated that practitioners should make every effort to exclude third-party observers during neuropsychological evaluations.[38] This guideline is based on a prior statement made by the APA that the presence of third-party observers in the testing room violates principles of standardized test administration, as set forth in their *Ethical Principles of Psychologists and Code of Conduct*, and concerns that neuropsychological test measures have not been standardized for the presence of these observers.[38] Misgivings have also arisen regarding "observer effect," whereby the presence of third parties may influence a testee's performance. Of note, the aforementioned position paper explicitly allows third-party observers in formal educational observation of trainees and parents without any distinguishing explanation as to the affect that these third-party observers might have. This distinction has not gone unnoticed and has been criticized.[39] A similar policy by the

AACN has been enunciated, limited to civil litigation.[40] In 2007, however, the APA significantly modified its stance on the presence of third-party observers, recognizing that these observations "may facilitate validity and fairness of the evaluation or be required by law."[41] Accordingly, the APA recommended the following options: (1) conduct the assessment in the presence of the third-party observer, but take appropriate steps to minimize any potential third-party observer effects (ie, seat the observer in a location so that the test taker cannot view the individual or obtain a commitment in advance that the observer will not speak or in any other way attempt to influence the examination); (2) minimize the intrusion, by taking steps designed to ensure that the observation takes place in the least intrusive fashion (ie, through a one way mirror or by audio or video taping the session); (3) use testing assessment measures that are less affected by observation; (4) take steps to protect the integrity of the testing process (ie, demanding that the request for third-party observation be withdrawn and seeking court intervention, if necessary, in an attempt to obtain a favorable ruling disallowing such observation); or (5) simply refusing to perform the examination, based on concerns regarding the integrity of the testing and resulting opinions if third-party observation is permitted. In each instance the choice is left to the judgment of the examiner, resulting in a professional state of chaos.

MALINGERING

Individuals claiming disability as a result of TBI are frequently confronted with accusations of malingering, exaggeration, and secondary gain, which must be addressed by the forensic evaluation. These issues are most frequently seen in cases of mild TBI. The use of these labels is tantamount to accusing the plaintiff of fabricating his or her claim. The suggestion of intentional falsehood and perhaps even perjury must be approached with extreme caution.

Malingering has been defined by the APA as the "intentional production of false or grossly exaggerated physical or psychological symptoms motivated by external incentives."[42] A battery of malingering "tests" have been formulated that can purportedly distinguish the malingerer from the legitimately injured individual. The implicit assumption is that a test can differentiate a person with a true brain injury from one feigning such symptoms and complaints. However, the supposition that a test can be constructed to achieve this goal ignores fundamental truths inherent in cases of TBI. If an individual is labeled as having a lack of motivation, is it because they are intentionally malingering, or is it due to the effects of traumatic brain damage itself? Individuals exhibiting mild TBI are often convinced that no one will believe them and therefore may tend to exaggerate their symptoms. Should failing the test be attributed to chronic pain and depression, or intentional falsehoods on the part of the test taker? The conclusion that one failed to use their best effort on these tests assumes that even brain-injured individuals have the capacity to consistently apply best efforts from task to task. Furthermore, the conclusion of malingering presumes that a person cannot have a brain injury regardless of their failing score on these examinations. This inappropriate assumption fails to assess with any degree of accuracy what percentage or portion of the injured victim's courtroom testimony is true or false.

While there are several malingering tests in existence, there is no single test that has achieved universal acceptance as the "gold standard" in determining whether an individual is malingering. A major criticism leveled against these tests is the absence of any studies comparing verified brain-injured individuals with those without brain injury. The study samples and the norms constructed from them improperly rely on test takers being instructed to feign malingering and their ability to implement these instructions.[26]

Although the NAN has accepted the use of symptom validity assessments "as a component of a medically necessary evaluation," and the AACN has reached a consensus that "clinicians can diagnose malingering in some examinees," there nevertheless remains considerable controversy in the neuropsychological field as to the use and validity of these evaluations.[43] As the AAN has noted, "there is no established neuropsychological profile diagnostic of malingering."[44] These tests, according to many, provide only limited and partial insight, and "neuropsychologists must be extremely judicious in their interpretation of the symptom validity test data. Test performance below recommended cutoffs is not a *sine qua non* of malingering."[10]

From the legal perspective, allowing an expert witness to formulate a conclusion about malingering invades the province of the jury or fact finder. The Court must serve as a sentinel and exclude opinions and testimony that are not generally accepted within the scientific community, are inherently unreliable, or have the capacity to prejudice or confuse the jury. This type of testimony incorrectly permits a witness to directly comment on another witness's credibility. Expert testimony is generally inadmissible where it relates solely to the issue of credibility.[45] In effect, malingering testimony has the same role as the lie detector, which places an imprimatur on the veracity of a witness. The introduction of lie detector results is prohibited in most jurisdictions.[46] Permissive use of opinions of malingering elicits justifiable fear that a jury may place too much credence on this type of testimony and forgo independent analysis of the other evidence presented.

This is not to suggest, however, that an objective assessment should ignore scientific reality. A forensic examiner certainly must identify atypical presentations, bizarre or absurd symptoms, atypical symptom fluctuation, and impossibly severe complaints of deficits. On the other hand, an objective assessment must also explore hypotheses for poor performance other than malingering. In all instances where malingering becomes a point of contention, a litigant is permitted to testify and explain his or her particular limitations and condition. In addition, the plaintiff is afforded the opportunity to introduce the testimony of third-party witnesses who have had the opportunity to observe the individual at home, at work, and within the community. The jury is always free to reject the opinion of any expert in favor of any or all of the other testimony introduced into evidence.

THE FAKE BAD SCALE AND ITS ROLE IN FORENSIC EVALUATIONS

Perhaps no area in the forensic evaluation of brain injury survivors provokes more controversy than the administration and analysis of the Fake Bad Scale (FBS), as part of the Minnesota Multiphasic Personality Inventory (MMPI-2). Although the MMPI is reportedly the most widely administered psychological test in the world,[47] its inclusion of the FBS scale in 2006 has provoked contentious debate in brain injury litigation.[48] The test has recently been renamed the symptom validity scale, to avoid the negative connotation that the former name aroused.[49] The scale requires an individual to respond "true" or "false" to 43 subjective statements concerning his or her health, and emotional and physical status. On the basis of a scaled score, Lees-Hailey and English[50] opine that symptom exaggeration and falsification can be detected. Critics of the scale, including James Butcher, one of the principal coinvestigators of the revised MMPI-2 norms, contend that "the scale is likely to classify an unacceptably large number of individuals who are experiencing genuine psychological distress as malingerers. It is recommended that the FBS not be used in clinical settings nor should it be used during disability evaluations."[51]

A brief review of the 43 true-false questions, quoted in a front-page Wall Street Journal story, such as "My sleep is fitful and disturbed," "I have nightmares every few nights," "I have very few headaches," "I have few or no pains," "There seems to be a lump in my throat much of the time," "Once a week or oftener, I suddenly feel hot all over, for no reason," "I have a great deal of stomach trouble," are statements that one might expect a person with brain damage, sleep disorders, headaches, post-traumatic stress disorder, depression, and/or anxiety to endorse.[48] The patient accumulates points for confirming the very symptoms characteristic of his or her condition. Critics further contend that the test has a bias against women.[52] Lees-Hailey and Fox[53] have set a cutoff score of 20 for men and 24 for women. The criticism leveled against the FBS has been characterized by test proponents as being "naïve and inaccurate" and "absurd."[53] While the publishers of the MMPI-2, University of Minnesota Press, still use and score the FBS, reportedly the APA Committee on Disability Issues in Psychology (CDIP), in a letter dated May 31, 2007, strongly recommended that an independent empirical evaluation of the FBS be conducted to determine the scale's validity.[54]

COVERING THE COST OF LONG-TERM BRAIN INJURY CARE

Persons suffering from TBI often require long-term care. This type of care is extremely expensive and often not covered by group health insurance, as insurance carriers categorize it as "rehabilitation" services rather than "acute medical care." When private coverage is provided it is often limited in duration, scope, and dollar amount, which frequently leads to less than optimal results for patients. In other instances future treatment is greatly curtailed, due to the failure to provide confirmation of immediate success in the established treatment plan. Where the cost of care is not an issue, such as the worker's compensation arena, or no-fault insurance and long-term care contracts, issues concerning the lack of evidence-based studies to substantiate the treatment sought, further complicates the process for gaining insurance company approval for long-term cognitive rehabilitation.

Long-term outcome studies confirm that the cognitive and emotional consequences of TBI are not related to the initial severity of brain injury. These impairments are amenable to intervention to minimize long-term disability even years later.[55] The failure of individuals to receive these services either because of a failure on the part of insurance carriers to authorize treatment, or the failure on the part of providers to make these services available, is equally troubling.

The Brain Injury Association of America, in an effort to illuminate the need for insurance reimbursement for the costs of long-term rehabilitation, has formulated a position paper that conceptualizes TBI as a long-term disease rather than the end result of a specific condition, and promotes the following principles in support.[56]

1. Brain injury is not an event or an outcome, "but a life-long **disease process** that impacts brain and body functions including physical, communication, cognitive and emotional skills." The reformulation of TBI as a disease process rather than an event or a final outcome attempts to remove issues of reimbursement from the traditional rehabilitation model and replace it with a long-term treatment model, necessitating long-term care.
2. A person with a brain injury requires an individualized treatment plan that provides for necessary treatment "that has a reasonable expectation of achieving

measurable functional improvements in a predictable period of time through the provision of treatment of sufficient scope, duration and intensity."

3. A person with a brain injury requires access to the "full treatment continuum to manage the disease" including acute and postacute treatment as both an inpatient and outpatient.

4. Treatment must be provided in the most appropriate treatment setting through accredited programs (including acute care hospitals, inpatient rehabilitation facilities, residential rehabilitation facilities, day treatment programs, outpatient clinics, and home health agencies).

5. Private insurance carriers must be prevented from inappropriately transferring the cost of care of those with brain injuries to the public sector.

Several insurance carriers have recently changed their policies regarding reimbursement for the long-term rehabilitation costs associated with brain trauma. One plan now recognizes cognitive rehabilitation as only being "medically necessary" in the treatment of patients with significantly impaired cognitive function following a TBI. However, this plan never fully defines what "significant" means in this context. The same plan deems cognitive rehabilitation following stroke, dementia, Parkinson disease, and anoxic brain injury still to be investigational, and not medically necessary. The allowable International Classification of Diseases codes for treatment are either skull fractures or intracranial injury, and do not include codes for concussion, mild TBI, or postconcussion syndrome.[57] This same carrier has imposed the requirement that following admission to a cognitive rehabilitation program, documentation of functional improvement within 2 to 4 weeks of admission must be produced before further treatment will be approved. This time constraint is simply an arbitrary period designed by an insurance carrier to limit or preclude coverage for legitimate and necessary care.

Another national health insurance carrier has modified its plan to provide coverage for cognitive rehabilitation following TBI, brain injury due to stroke, aneurysm, anoxia, encephalitis, brain tumors, and brain toxins, when the patient can actively participate. This carrier still considers cognitive rehabilitation to be unproven for cerebral palsy, Down syndrome, Alzheimer disease, attention deficit disorder, and developmental disorders such autism and Parkinson disease. In addition, the carrier contends that coma stimulation remains an unproven modality of treatment for comatose or minimally responsive patients.[58]

The scientific justification for long-term cognitive, behavioral, and physical rehabilitation following a brain injury remains a matter of considerable controversy, fueling the insurance industry's reluctance to pay for the costs associated with this type of care. In 1999, a US National Institutes of Health (NIH) Consensus Panel was formed to examine the efficacy of brain injury rehabilitation. The consensus panel reviewed the medical literature from January 1988 through August 1998 regarding cognitive and behavioral therapy following all forms of TBI, and concluded that although there was evidence of documented success, further research regarding effectiveness was necessary.[59]

Since the initial recommendations of the NIH Consensus Panel there have been other attempts to establish evidence-based recommendations for rehabilitation following an acquired brain injury. Unfortunately, however, there have been few class I studies on which to formulate recommendations. Based on a review of all available class I, II, and III studies, the investigators concurred that further research is still necessary, but nonetheless concluded that substantial evidence does exist to support cognitive rehabilitation for individuals suffering from TBI including strategy training for mild memory impairments, strategy training for postacute attention deficits, and interventions for functional communication deficits.[60]

The recent passage of national health care reform legislation (The Patient Protection and Affordable Care Act HR 3590) has favorable implications for the treatment continuum for persons with TBI. The Act authorizes the Secretary of Health and Human Services to define the essential health care package of benefits available to all citizens. The Act specifically lists benefits for: (1) rehabilitative and habilitative services and devices, (2) mental health and substance use disorder services, including behavioral treatment, and (3) chronic disease management. According to the *Statement of Understanding Regarding Coverage of the Treatment Continuum for Persons with Brain Injury Under this Act*, placed in the Congressional record by Congressman Bill Pascrell, Jr in his capacity as cochair of the Congressional Traumatic Brain Injury Task Force (March 22, 2010), "the term 'rehabilitative and habilitative services' includes items and services used to restore functional capacity, minimize limitations on physical and cognitive functions, and maintain or prevent deterioration of functioning as a result of an illness, injury, disorder or other health condition. Such services also include training of individuals with mental and physical disabilities to enhance functional development."

The Act further provides that the benefits approved under the essential benefit package should be made in accordance with generally accepted standards of medical and other appropriate clinical or professional practice, and without restriction that cannot be attributable to critical appropriateness. According to the aforesaid understanding, "consistent with medical, clinical and professional practice, appropriateness should be determined based upon the unique needs of the individual with brain injury and treatment should be of sufficient scope, duration and intensity."

It is hoped that with the implementation of this landmark legislation, all citizens suffering from TBI will be able to obtain the full array of services and products to facilitate their ability to maintain and improve their function and quality of life.

SUMMARY

By virtue of the traumatic causes of brain injury, law and medicine are inextricably intertwined. The medical profession has and will continue to play a crucial role in the courtroom when cases of brain injury are litigated. Similarly, jurisprudence will continue to have an influence on the ways that scientific beliefs are tested and the opinions that are derived from these beliefs in the field of brain trauma.

REFERENCES

1. Faul M, Xu L, Wald MM, et al. Traumatic brain injury in the United States: emergency department visits, hospitalizations and deaths 2002–2006. Atlanta (GA): Centers for Disease Control and Prevention, National Center for Injury Prevention and Control; 2010.
2. Corrigan J, Selassie A, Orman J. The epidemiology of traumatic brain injury. J Head Trauma Rehabil 2010;25:72–80.
3. Available at: http://www.uscourts.gov/rules/Evidence_Rules_2007.pdf. Accessed April 23, 2010.
4. Williams MA, Mackin GA, Beresford HR, et al. Qualifications and guidelines for the physician expert witness. Neurology 2006;66:13–4.
5. Lezak M, Howieson D, Loring D. Neuropsychological assessment. New York: Oxford University Press; 2004.

6. Herman S. Report of the therapeutics and technology assessment subcommittee of the American Academy of Neurology. Neurology 1996;47:592–9.

7. American Academy of Clinical Neuropsychology. Practice guidelines for neuropsychological assessment and consultation. Clin Neuropsychol 2007;21:209–31.

8. Bigler E, Brooks M. Traumatic brain injury and forensic neuropsychology. J Head Trauma Rehabil 2009;24:76–87.

9. Ethical principles of psychologists and code of conduct, 9.01(b). Available at: http://www.apa.org/ethics/code2002.html. Accessed April 23, 2010.

10. Herman S. Report of the therapeutics and technology assessment subcommittee of the American Academy of Neurology, assessment: neuropsychological testing of adults. Considerations for neurologists. Neurology 1966;47:592–9.

11. Adamson v Chiovaro, 308 NJ. Super 70, 1998.

12. Johns v Im, 263 Va 315, 2002.

13. Combs v Norfolk and Western Rwy. Co, 256 Va 490, 1998.

14. Steinbuch v Stern 2 AD3d 709, 4th Department, 2003.

15. Frye v US, 293 F, 1013.

16. Daubert v Merrell Dow, 509 US 579 See, Federal rule of evidence 702 adapting the Daubert standard in all federal courts.

17. Wood R. The scientist-practitioner model: how do advances in clinical and cognitive neuroscience affect neuropsychology in the courtroom? J Head Trauma Rehabil 2009;24:88–99.

18. Sweet JJ, Mosberg PJ, Suchy Y. Ten-year follow-up survey of clinical neuropsychologists: part I. Practices and beliefs. Clin Neuropsychol 2000;15:301–9.

19. Sweet JJ, Peck E, Abromowitx C, et al. National Academy of Neuropsychology/Division 40 of the American Psychological Association practice survey of clinical neuropsychology in the United States, Part 1: practitioner and practice characteristics, professional activities, time requirements. Clin Neuropsychol 2002;16:109–27.

20. Ruff RM, Iverson GL, Barth JT, et al. Recommendations for diagnosing a mild traumatic brain injury: a National academy of neuropsychology education paper. Arch Clin Neuropsychol 2009;24:3–10.

21. McCrea M, Pliskin N, Barth J, et al. Official position of the military TBI task force on the role of neuropsychology and rehabilitation psychology in the evaluation, management, and research of military veterans with traumatic brain injury. Clin Neuropsychol 2008;22:10–26.

22. Powell JM, Ferraro JV, Dikman SS, et al. Accuracy of mild traumatic brain injury diagnosis. Arch Phys Med Rehabil 2008;89:1550–5.

23. Coleman M, Davis M, Rodd J. Towards the routine use of brain imaging to aid the clinical disorders of disorders of consciousness. Brain 2009;132:2541–52.

24. Giancio J, Ashwal N, Childs R, et al. The minimally conscious state: definition and diagnostic criteria. Neurology 2002;58:349–53.

25. McDougald v Garber, 73 NY2d 246; New York court of appeals, 1989.

26. Zasler N, Katz D, Zafonte R. Brain injury medicine principles and practice. New York (NY): Demo Press; 2007. p. 423.

27. Giacino J, Whyte J. The vegetative and minimally conscious states: current knowledge and remaining questions. J Head Trauma Rehabil 2005;20:30–50.

28. Giacino J, Smart C. Recent advances in behavioral assessment of individuals with disorders of consciousness. Curr Opin Neurol 2007;20:614–9.

29. Pike v Honseinger, 155 NY 201.

30. Jagoda A, Bazarian J, Bruns J, et al. Clinical policy: neuroimaging and decision making in adult mild traumatic brain injury in the acute setting clinical. Ann Emerg Med 2008;52:714–48.

31. Federal rule of evidence, 803(18).
32. Hinlickly v Dreyfuss, 6 NY3d 636 (New York Court of Appeals, 2006).
33. Ponce v Health Ins. Plan of Greater NY, 100 A.D.2d 963 (2nd Deptartment 1984) and Bazakos v Lewis, 56 AD2d 15 (2nd Dept. 2008).
34. Pennsylvania Rules of Civil Procedure 4010.
35. Zimbler v Resnick 72nd street Associates, 876 N.Y.S.2d 18, 1st Dept. 2009.
36. Jessica H. ex rel. Arp v Spagnola. 41 A.D.3d 1261, 839 N.Y.S.2d 638; 4th Dept. 2007.
37. National Academy of Neuropsychology. Presence of third party observers during neuropsychological testing. Arch Clin Neuropsychol 2000;15:379–80.
38. American Psychological Association. Ethical principles of psychologists and code of conduct. Am Psychol 1992;47:1597–1161.
39. Otto R, Kraus D. Contemplating the presence of third party observers and facilitators in psychological evaluations. Assessment 2009;16:362–72.
40. American Academy of Clinical Neuropsychology. Policy statement on the presence of third party observers in neuropsychological assessments. Clin Neuropsychol 2001;15:433–9.
41. American Psychological Association. Committee on psychological tests and assessment. Statement on third party observers in psychological testing and assessment: a framework for decision making. Available at: http://www.apa.org/science/programs/testing/third-party-observers.pdf. Accessed April 23, 2010.
42. American Psychiatric Association. DSM-IV-TR, diagnostic and statistical manual of mental disorders. 4th edition. Arlington (VA): American Psychiatric Association; 2000. p. 739. Text Revision.
43. Bush SS, Ruff RM, Troster AL, et al. Symptom validity assessment: practice issues and medical necessity NAN policy and planning committee. Arch Clin Neuropsychol 2005;20:419–26.
44. Heilbronner RL. American academy of clinical neuropsychology consensus conference statement on the neuropsychological assessment of effort, response bias, and malingering. Clin Neuropsychol 2009;23:1093–129.
45. Ruff R. Best practice guidelines for forensic neuropsychological examinations of patients with traumatic brain injury. J Head Trauma Rehabil 2009;24:131–40.
46. People v Shedrick, 66 NY2d 1015.
47. Pope K, Butcher J, Seeley J. The MMPI, MMPI2 and MMPIA in court. 3rd edition. Arlington (VA): American Psychological Association; 2006. p. 7.
48. Armstrong D. Malingering roils personal-injury law. Wall Street Journal. March 5, 2008;1:A12.
49. Ben-Porath Y, Tellegen A, Graham J. The MMPI-2 symptom validity scale. Minneapolis (MN): University of Minnesota Press; 2008.
50. Lees-Haley P, English GW. A fake bad scale on the MMPI-2 for personal injury claimants. Psychol Rep 1991;68:203–10.
51. Butcher JN, Arbisi PA, Atlis MM, et al. The construct validity of the Lees-Haley Fake Bad Scale: does this scale measure somatic malingering and feigned emotional distress? Arch Clin Neuropsychol 2008;23:855 64.
52. Lees-Hailey P. Efficacy of MMPI-II validity scale and MCM1-II modifiers scales for detecting spurious PTSD claims; F, F-K, fake bad scale, ego strength, subtle obvious subscales, DIS and DEB. J Clin Psychol 1992;48:681–9.
53. Lees-Haley PR, Fox DD. Commentary on butcher, Arbisi, Atlis and McNulty (2003) on the fake bad scale. Arch Clin Neuropsychol 2004;19:33–336.

54. Gass CS, Williams CL, Cumella E, et al. Ambiguous measures of unknown constructs: the MMPI-2 fake bad scale (aka symptom validity scale, FBS, FBS-r). Psychol Inj Law 2010;3(1):81–5.

55. Whitall L, Mcmillan TM, Murray GD, et al. Disability in young people and adults after head injury: 5-7 year follow up of a prospective cohort study. J Neurol Neurosurg Psychiatr 2006;77:640–5.

56. Conceptualizing Brain Injury as a Chronic Disease. Position paper of the brain injury association of America. March 2009. Available at: http://www.biausa.org/elements/pdfs/position_chronic_disease_mar_2009.pdf. Accessed April 24, 2010.

57. Anthem-blue cross-blue shield Policy No. MED.0081 effective 10/22/2008.

58. United Health Care Network Bulletin, Vol. 31 May 2009, Medical policy updates revised policies can be reviewed on line at: UnitedHealthCareOnline.com>Tools & Resources>Policies and Protocols>Medical Policies.

59. NIH Consensus development panel on rehabilitation of persons with traumatic brain injury. Rehabilitation of persons with traumatic brain injury. JAMA 1999; 282:974–83.

60. Cicerone K, Dahlberg M, Malec J, et al. Evidence-based cognitive rehabilitation: updated review of literature from 1998-2002. Arch Phys Med Rehabil 2005;86: 1681–92.

Index

Note: Page numbers of article titles are in **boldface** type.

Psychiatr Clin N Am 33 (2010) 931–940
doi:10.1016/S0193-953X(10)00088-2
0193-953X/10/$ – see front matter © 2010 Elsevier Inc. All rights reserved.

psych.theclinics.com

United States Postal Service

Statement of Ownership, Management, and Circulation
(All Periodicals Publications Except Requestor Publications)

1. Publication Title	2. Publication Number									3. Filing Date
Psychiatric Clinics of North America	0	0	0		7	0	3			9/15/10

4. Issue Frequency	5. Number of Issues Published Annually	6. Annual Subscription Price
Mar, Jun, Sep, Dec	4	$248.00

7. Complete Mailing Address of Known Office of Publication (Not printer) (Street, city, county, state, and ZIP+4®)

Elsevier Inc.
360 Park Avenue South
New York, NY 10010-1710

Contact Person
Stephen Bushing
Telephone (Include area code)
215-239-3688

8. Complete Mailing Address of Headquarters or General Business Office of Publisher (Not printer)

Elsevier Inc., 360 Park Avenue South, New York, NY 10010-1710

9. Full Names and Complete Mailing Addresses of Publisher, Editor, and Managing Editor (Do not leave blank)

Publisher (Name and complete mailing address)

Kim Murphy, Elsevier, Inc., 1600 John F. Kennedy Blvd. Suite 1800, Philadelphia, PA 19103-2899

Editor (Name and complete mailing address)

Sarah Barth, Elsevier, Inc., 1600 John F. Kennedy Blvd. Suite 1800, Philadelphia, PA 19103-2899

Managing Editor (Name and complete mailing address)

Catherine Bewick, Elsevier, Inc., 1600 John F. Kennedy Blvd. Suite 1800, Philadelphia, PA 19103-2899

10. Owner (Do not leave blank. If the publication is owned by a corporation, give the name and address of the corporation immediately followed by the names and addresses of all stockholders owning or holding 1 percent or more of the total amount of stock. If not owned by a corporation, give the names and addresses of the individual owners. If owned by a partnership or other unincorporated firm, give its name and address as well as those of each individual owner. If the publication is published by a nonprofit organization, give its name and address.)

Full Name	Complete Mailing Address
Wholly owned subsidiary of	4520 East-West Highway
Reed/Elsevier, US holdings	Bethesda, MD 20814

11. Known Bondholders, Mortgagees, and Other Security Holders Owning or Holding 1 Percent or More of Total Amount of Bonds, Mortgages, or Other Securities. If none, check box → ☐ None

Full Name	Complete Mailing Address
N/A	

12. Tax Status (For completion by nonprofit organizations authorized to mail at nonprofit rates) (Check one)
The purpose, function, and nonprofit status of this organization and the exempt status for federal income tax purposes:
☐ Has Not Changed During Preceding 12 Months
☐ Has Changed During Preceding 12 Months (Publisher must submit explanation of change with this statement)

PS Form 3526, September 2007 (Page 1 of 3 (Instructions Page 3)) PSN 7530-01-000-9931 PRIVACY NOTICE: See our Privacy policy in www.usps.com

---

13. Publication Title			14. Issue Date for Circulation Data Below
Psychiatric Clinics of North America			September 2010

15. Extent and Nature of Circulation			Average No. Copies Each Issue During Preceding 12 Months	No. Copies of Single Issue Published Nearest to Filing Date
a. Total Number of Copies (Net press run)			1473	1400
b. Paid Circulation (By Mail and Outside the Mail)	(1)	Mailed Outside-County Paid Subscriptions Stated on PS Form 3541. (Include paid distribution above nominal rate, advertiser's proof copies, and exchange copies)	730	654
	(2)	Mailed In-County Paid Subscriptions Stated on PS Form 3541 (Include paid distribution above nominal rate, advertiser's proof copies, and exchange copies)		
	(3)	Paid Distribution Outside the Mails Including Sales Through Dealers and Carriers, Street Vendors, Counter Sales, and Other Paid Distribution Outside USPS®	265	280
	(4)	Paid Distribution by Other Classes Mailed Through the USPS (e.g. First-Class Mail®)		
c. Total Paid Distribution (Sum of 15b (1), (2), (3), and (4))		▶	995	934
d. Free or Nominal Rate Distribution (By Mail and Outside the Mail)	(1)	Free or Nominal Rate Outside-County Copies Included on PS Form 3541	84	63
	(2)	Free or Nominal Rate In-County Copies Included on PS Form 3541		
	(3)	Free or Nominal Rate Copies Mailed at Other Classes Through the USPS (e.g. First-Class Mail)		
	(4)	Free or Nominal Rate Distribution Outside the Mail (Carriers or other means)		
e. Total Free or Nominal Rate Distribution (Sum of 15d (1), (2), (3) and (4))		▶	84	63
f. Total Distribution (Sum of 15c and 15e)		▶	1079	997
g. Copies not Distributed (See instructions to publishers #4 (page #3))		▶	394	403
h. Total (Sum of 15f and g)		▶	1473	1400
i. Percent Paid (15c divided by 15f times 100)			92.22%	93.68%

16. Publication of Statement of Ownership

☐ If the publication is a general publication, publication of this statement is required. Will be printed in the December 2010 issue of this publication.   ☐ Publication not required

17. Signature and Title of Editor, Publisher, Business Manager, or Owner

Stephen R. Bushing

Stephen R. Bushing – Fulfillment/Inventory Specialist   Date September 15, 2010

I certify that all information furnished on this form is true and complete. I understand that anyone who furnishes false or misleading information on this form or who omits material or information requested on the form may be subject to criminal sanctions (including fines and imprisonment) and/or civil sanctions (including civil penalties).

PS Form 3526, September 2007 (Page 2 of 3)

Moving?

Make sure your subscription moves with you!

To notify us of your new address, find your **Clinics Account Number** (located on your mailing label above your name), and contact customer service at:

Email: journalscustomerservice-usa@elsevier.com

800-654-2452 (subscribers in the U.S. & Canada)
314-447-8871 (subscribers outside of the U.S. & Canada)

Fax number: 314-447-8029

Elsevier Health Sciences Division
Subscription Customer Service
3251 Riverport Lane
Maryland Heights, MO 63043

*To ensure uninterrupted delivery of your subscription, please notify us at least 4 weeks in advance of move.

Printed and bound by CPI Group (UK) Ltd, Croydon, CR0 4YY

03/10/2024

01040456-0001